Marta Regina Pinheiro Flores
Carlos E. P. Machado
Ricardo H. A. da Silva

Proposal for photoanthropometric frontal facial analysis

Marta Regina Pinheiro Flores
Carlos E. P. Machado
Ricardo H. A. da Silva

Proposal for photoanthropometric frontal facial analysis

Descriptive methodology of anatomical reference points

ScienciaScripts

Imprint
Any brand names and product names mentioned in this book are subject to trademark, brand or patent protection and are trademarks or registered trademarks of their respective holders. The use of brand names, product names, common names, trade names, product descriptions etc. even without a particular marking in this work is in no way to be construed to mean that such names may be regarded as unrestricted in respect of trademark and brand protection legislation and could thus be used by anyone.

Cover image: www.ingimage.com

This book is a translation from the original published under ISBN 978-3-330-76461-3.

Publisher:
Sciencia Scripts
is a trademark of
Dodo Books Indian Ocean Ltd. and OmniScriptum S.R.L publishing group

120 High Road, East Finchley, London, N2 9ED, United Kingdom
Str. Armeneasca 28/1, office 1, Chisinau MD-2012, Republic of Moldova, Europe
Managing Directors: Ieva Konstantinova, Victoria Ursu
info@omniscriptum.com

Printed at: see last page
ISBN: 978-620-8-50501-1

DEDICATORY

I dedicate this work

To my family, who have always been by my side, especially my grandmother Delivina Custódio de Jesuz.

To my parents Marco Antônio Pereira Flores and Tânia Regina Pinheiro Flores, for their example of life and for supporting my choices and encouraging me to pursue my goals. You are the reason for my endeavours.

To my siblings Marco Antônio Pinheiro Flores and Mara Cristina Pinheiro Flores, for being part of my life and for understanding my absence at important times in their lives.

To my love, partner and friend, Helder Wilhan Blaskievicz, for his unconditional affection and understanding, supporting, encouraging and advising me at every moment of this labourious journey. You were largely responsible for this achievement in my life.

To my dear professor, Carlos Eduardo Palhares Machado, for the friendship he built, for the knowledge he passed on, for following every stage of this work and making it possible for this dream to come true.

Without each of these people, none of this would have come true.

ACKNOWLEDGEMENTS

To SEPAEL, the Audiovisual and Electronic Forensics Service of the National Institute of Criminalistics of the Federal Police, in the person of the head of the service and Federal Criminal Expert, André Luiz da Costa Morisson, for providing the software used in this study and for authorising my access to the 6th Facial Recognition Course of the National Police Academy (ANP), a course which has made a fundamental contribution to my learning.

To Gustavo Henrique Machado de Arruda, professor of the 6th Facial Recognition Course and Federal Criminal Expert, for the knowledge he imparted and for being so welcoming at every stage of this work.

To Federal Police Clerk Edmar Antônio da Silva for contributing his knowledge to make the software used in the study feasible and for always being willing to contribute.

To the Oral Rehabilitation Programme of the Faculty of Dentistry of Ribeirão Preto - USP, in the person of the coordinator, Professor Fernanda de Carvalho Panzeri Pires de Souza, who sometimes comforted me in difficult moments.

CAPES, for the financial support that allowed me to dedicate myself exclusively to this work.

PRESENTATION

In view of the lack of standardisation and objectivity in facial analysis of frontal images, the aim was to re-adapt the classic cephalometric descriptions in the literature, inserting visual references for their indirect application, thus favouring facial examination based exclusively on images. The adapted descriptions, known as photoanthropometrics, aim to provide the scientific, police and forensic community with more objective methodological aids for forensic facial analysis. This is a circumstance that is commonly demanded in the forensic routine in comparative processes of Forensic Facial Identification.

This paper is the result of a dissertation submitted to the Ribeirão Preto School of Dentistry at the University of São Paulo to obtain a Master's degree in the Oral Rehabilitation Postgraduate Programme in 2014.

SUMMARY

CHAPTER 1

Introduction

1.1. The *Human Face*

The face is the part of the body that most synthesises the human being, containing structures that are studied by the most diverse areas of science. Information related to an individual's beauty, appearance and health, as well as their emotions, can be gathered by simply analysing their structures visually (TAYLOR, 2001). Because it contains a large concentration of information-receiving organs (sense organs - sight, hearing, smell, taste and touch), the human face functions as a veritable centre for sending and receiving information, and is considered one of man's most important social tools. This tool significantly influences interpersonal relationships and the behaviour an individual establishes with the environment in which they live (ALLEY, 1998; EKMAN; FRIESEN, 2003). It is the main means of everyday interpersonal recognition, enabling individuals to routinely relate to each other without the need for a system that formally identifies them (ENLOW, 1990; HENNESSY; MOSS, 2001; WILKINSON, 2008).

Facial analyses are commonly carried out to obtain useful information for the most diverse fields of science, from art to science, such as sculpture, painting, architecture, anatomy, anthropometry and orthodontics. Art science studies the face in order to understand beauty, so that artists can create their paintings and sculptures according to the facial proportions of a particular group or aesthetic standard (GEORGE, 2007). In the scientific field, facial analyses are carried out in a variety of studies and for the most diverse purposes, such as: gathering information about a given population; obtaining craniofacial development and growth patterns to study the normality of a population for industrial purposes, for the development of tools and equipment for leisure and sport, as well as for the development of police and military equipment; early diagnosis of anomalies, delays in craniofacial development and syndromic facial characteristics (ALLANSON et al., 2011; ALVES, 2008; FARKAS; DEUTSCH, 1996; MUTSVANGWA; DOUGLAS, 2007); planning clinical and surgical, aesthetic or reconstructive interventions (FARKAS; DEUTSCH, 1996; PHAM; TOLLEFSON, 2010; STEVENS; CALHOUN; QUINN, 1997); studying and assessing facial aesthetics

(KUNJUR; SABESAN; ILANKOVAN, 2006), as well as its attractiveness (RHODES et al., 1998; RHODES, 2006).

The main purpose of scientific facial analyses is to search for patterns, whether of variation, association, causality or inheritance, in order to study the probability of occurrence of a certain characteristic in the sample studied (DEMAYO et al., 2009). By examining biological variation between populations, it is possible to obtain valuable information about the mechanisms of change and the evolutionary process of various groups over time (JURMAIN; KILGORE; TREVANTHAN, 2009). In scientific analysis, therefore, unlike artistic analyses, "how it should be" is less interesting and "how it is" is more important (MACHADO et al., 2014). This information is extremely important for forensic sciences, more specifically in classification methodologies (individual inclusion and exclusion within population groups) for human identification purposes (MACHADO et al., 2014).

The breadth of areas that depend on or have the face as their object of study shows the importance of developing and establishing facial analysis methodologies for understanding the population under study. Regardless of the area of interest, the definition, standardisation and validation of scientific methodologies contribute to the reproducibility of studies in different centres, allowing the resulting information to be compared in order to produce coherent, reliable and representative data. As this is an area that requires greater scientific rigour in its analyses, this work establishes a greater connection with issues involving forensic application, since facial structures are routinely used to survey population anthropometric patterns in biotypological studies and traces for age estimation, ancestry and gender determination, as well as for the establishment and standardisation of facial identification and recognition techniques.

1.2. Facial Analysis

Interest in anatomy and body and facial proportions dates back to the beginning of human civilisation (VALE, 2004; VEGTER; HAGE, 2000) and, contrary to what one might imagine, anthropometry, the term used to describe the study of measuring the human body for the purposes of classification and comparison (TAYLOR et al., 1993), has its origins not in medicine, nor in biology, but in the arts, being first used in the ancient civilisations of India, Egypt and Greece (PETROSKI, 1995).

In the beginning, analyses of the shape and configuration of the human body, including the face, were carried out essentially through observation, in what is known as morphological analysis. Over time, precepts of proportionality, symmetry and geometry were inserted into the concept of "human beauty", inspiring artists to look for instruments to measure the body and face (IVERSEN; SHIBATA, 1975; VALE, 2004). The first tools used as reference measures were the parts of the human body themselves, such as the middle finger, the height of the head, the foot, the arm and the inch (PETROSKI, 1995). Although they are still used today, over time there was a need to develop more refined measurement techniques (PETROSKI, 1995; VALE, 2004).

During the Renaissance, the German artist Albrecht Durer (1417-1518) and the Italian Leonardo da Vinci (1452-1519) were the first to use vertical and horizontal anatomical points and tracings to establish methods for analysing facial alterations and asymmetries (VALE, 2004). In the area of human identification, Alphonse Bertillon (18531914) was the criminologist who initially developed anthropometry methodologies and, although they were developed for judicial purposes, they ended up contributing greatly to the development of anthropometry methodologies in general (HESS, 2010). Currently, researchers present and discuss different facial analysis techniques as a whole (ALLANSON et al., 2011; EKMAN; FRIESEN, 2003; ENLOW; HANS, 1996; RAMANATHAN; CHELLAPPA, 2006; RHODES et al., 2008; STEVENS; CALHOUN; QUINN, 1997; ZIMBLER; HAM, 2005).

Some areas of activity require the establishment of a rigid and systematic approach, while others only require recognising or noticing facial abnormalities. The vast majority of systematic facial analysis techniques rely on the use of anatomical reference points, an area of study in Physical Anthropology, more specifically Anthropometry. When this is carried out on the skull and face, the area of study is said to be Craniofacial Anthropometry.

1.3. Anthropometry as a Scientific Method

Anthropology can be simply defined as the study of humanity (JURMAIN, 2009). The word Anthropology is derived from the Greek words anthropos, meaning "human", and *logos,* meaning "word" or "study" (JURMAIN; KILGORE; TREVANTHAN, 2009). It is the field of research that studies human culture and the evolutionary aspects of its biology, from cultural, anthropological, archaeological, linguistic and physical or biological perspectives (JURMAIN; KILGORE; TREVANTHAN, 2009). In so-called *Physical* or *Biological Anthropology*, human physical variation is reflected upon and described in an attempt to explain the biological differences present between populations (JURMAIN; KILGORE; TREVANTHAN, 2009). Over time, it has played a fundamental role, especially in the development and application of quantitative methods, studied by Anthropometry.

Anthropometry, in turn, can be defined as the science of measuring body size (NASA, 1978). The word *Anthropometry* derives from the Greek *anthropos*, meaning "man", and *metrikos*, meaning "measure" (LUZ, 2011). It is a branch of the biological sciences whose aims are to study the measurable characteristics of human morphology and to quantitatively analyse the dimensional variations of the human body using measuring instruments (SOBRAL, 1985). It is a simple, low-cost, non-invasive technique that does not generate risks for the individual being analysed.

Despite the diversity of anthropometric applications in people's daily lives, the method has a large margin of error and is the subject of several studies to understand and control it. In general, when anthropometric measurements are repeated, variability can occur as a result of the diversity of the physical characteristics of the population being analysed, due to biological variation itself, which cannot be avoided, or due to variations in technique, which in turn can be avoided (PERINI et al., 2005).

The variability in anthropometric measurements caused by inconsistencies in the execution of the technique is responsible for a higher incidence of error (PERINI et al., 2005). In order to guarantee greater precision and improvement in the execution of analysis techniques, examiners need to master the methods used, as well as standardising the measuring instruments, the measurements themselves and the anatomical reference points (SANTOS; FURJÃO, 2003). This standardisation is necessary so that data from a given population can be collected through studies and research into its "normality", thus allowing the probability of a given characteristic occurring and the probability of compatibility with the standard to be calculated. This data contributes significantly to substantiating cases of human identification using images, as will be described below.

1.4. Craniofacial Anthropometry

Craniofacial anthropometry is the science of systematically measuring and quantitatively analysing dimensional variations in the skull and face (MORECROFT; FIELLER; EVISON, 2010). Until recently, this process was carried out manually, directly on the visible or palpable structures of the individual, by anthropometrists. However, with the development of new technologies, such as the discovery of X-rays by Wilhelm Konrad Roentgen in 1895, computerised tomography and magnetic resonance imaging in the 1980s and the increase in the number of image-producing devices, there has been a growing demand for indirect analyses, and with this, the need for alternative methodologies to direct measurement (MORECROFT; FIELLER; EVISON, 2010).

Regardless of whether the anthropometric analysis technique is direct or indirect, or whether the analysis system is manual or automated, in order for comparative processes in craniofacial anthropometry to be established, the determination of anatomical reference points is inevitable (MORECROFT; FIELLER; EVISON, 2010). These are called craniometric when restricted to the skull, and prosopometric or cephalometric when restricted to the face (ARBENZ, 1988). As the face is closely linked to the adjacent bone anatomy, many points initially defined in craniometry were transferred to cephalometric application (ARBENZ, 1988).

Anthropometric points can generally be categorised as: Type I or anatomical, positioned at the meeting of two varieties of tissues or structures; Type II or structural, geometrically defined at the maximum contour of a structure, such as those positioned at the most lateral points of the wings of the nose (for example, the Alar point); Type III or external, belonging to curves or surfaces, whose locations are defined according to the geometric characteristics of neighbouring anatomical structures (SFORZA et al., 2009). With the introduction of digital anthropometry, pseudo-points emerged, interposed between those already known, contributing to the contour of a surface and a broader assessment of the structure of interest (SFORZA et al., 2009).

Cephalometry, first described by Holly Broadbent (1894-1977), is an area of analysis in Craniofacial Anthropometry and consists of the study of head and neck measurements (HALL; GRIPP; SLAVOTINEK, 2006; SANTOS; FURJÃO, 2003). It is a resource used to quantify, classify, compare and communicate quantitative data on dentocraniofacial morphology by means of teleradiographs, and is mainly used in orthodontics to analyse the growth and development of these structures (CARDOSO et al., 2005). Because it was originally developed for use on radiographs, Cephalometry's descriptive basis for its anatomical reference points are the structures that can be visualised on radiographic images, which ends up hindering its determination when used on photographic images (VEGTER; HAGE, 2000).

Cephalometric analysis consists of collecting a set of angular, linear or proportional values, the bases of which are similar for different professionals, despite the different approaches given to metric information (WIERZBICKI, 2011). Artists use cephalometric information to create their paintings and sculptures; orthodontists and oral and maxillofacial surgeons use it to guide the changes they make to facial bones and teeth; similarly, anthropologists and forensic professionals use it to understand the characteristics that make a person different from others, such as a human identification protocol (MACHADO et al., 2014).

The anatomical reference points needed to establish linear and angular measurements can be classified as odd or median (as they are located on the median sagittal plane), or even, located on lateral planes (MACHADO et al., 2014). Farkas (1994) proposed and described a system of 47 anatomical points and a set of 132 head and face measurements, 103 of which were linear and 29 angular. He also proposed 155 facial indices and proportions that are still widely used today to describe the human face. Most of the cephalometric points were defined so that they could be visualised in frontal, lateral or base of nose views, or by palpating the underlying bone structures (FARKAS; DEUTSCH, 1996). Farkas is considered to be the most important influence on modern facial soft tissue anthropometry, contributing more than 120 publications in establishing standards for almost all facial and head soft tissue measurements (FARKAS, 1994; FARKAS; MUNRO, 1987).

Cephalometry, like anthropometry in general, has been the subject of several studies in an attempt to analyse and quantify the errors inherent to it. Systematic errors are those resulting from the magnification and distortion of radiographic images; random errors are those caused by the examiner visually inspecting the anatomical reference points on the radiograph (WIERZBICKI, 2011). The latter can be reduced by automating the determination of these anatomical structures and the measuring instruments (COHEN; LINNEY, 1984).

Regardless of the science that uses them and the substrate used to analyse them, individual perception and interpretation in defining these anatomical points are largely responsible for errors in their identification and in the angular and linear measurements taken from them (FARKAS; DEUTSCH, 1996; LAU; COOKE;

HÀGG, 1997). The observer's experience is an important factor in reducing errors in the variations of cephalometric measurements in relation to their averages. For this reason, training and calibration significantly reduces the errors made, but does not guarantee total reliability of the measurement methods (ALBUQUERQUE; ALMEIDA, 1998; LAU; COOKE; HÀGG, 1997; MARTINS et al., 1995; WIERZBICKI, 2011).

The use of indices and angles - rather than linear measurements - reduces the chance of error in measurements, as the values generally remain constant, regardless of magnification factors (SFORZA, 2009; WIERZBICKI, 2011). These tools can be used to eliminate potential differences between camera distances, thus allowing different images to be compared quantitatively (MORETON; MORLEY, 2011). They are indicated when there is a need to express shape rather than size, reveal one facial dimension as a percentage of another, or when comparing facial images of different sizes (HENNEBERG; SIMPSON; STEPHAN, 2003). In the age determination study by Ramanathan and Chellappa (2006), however, it was noted that only linear measurements should be taken, as angular measurements and tangential measurements of the face cannot be accurately estimated when analysing frontal facial images.

Another major problem with cephalometric image studies is that most of them use lateral projections, which makes them unsuitable for a large part of the world's scientific demand, especially in the area of forensic facial identification and recognition, which generally uses frontal facial images from civil and criminal identification records as a basis for comparison.

1.5. Facial Images for Human Identification Purposes

Capitalist development, culminating in the Industrial Revolution that began in England in the 18th century, completely changed the way millions of people lived and, from the 19th century onwards, it became necessary to create reliable identification systems that would make it possible to identify individuals who committed crimes and went against public order, unlike the method used until then, which was limited to personal names (SCORSATO, 2012). The creation of these systems would act to identify repeat offenders in particular, given that the stigmatising and mutilating penalties used at the time had recently been abolished (GINZBURG, 1989).

The invention of photography was the result of an arduous and long process of isolated discoveries by various artists, scientists and historians, who contributed knowledge of basic principles (such as the pinhole darkroom, photosensitivity and optics) that eventually culminated in the discovery of photography in its current form (HARRELL, 2002). The most important names in this process were the Frenchmen Joseph Nicéphore Niépce and Louis Jacques Mandé Daguerre, who contributed, respectively, to the production of the first permanent photograph in history, in 1826, and to the presentation of the first practical process of taking photographs, in 1839 (HARRELL, 2002). Since then, photography has been defined as an instrument of great documentary power and evidentiary capacity, as well as being a non-invasive and low-cost method for assessing facial tissues (SFORZA, 2009). These characteristics ended up making it one of the most important instruments in science (FABRIS, 2002). In police identification, the invention of photography was as important to criminology as the invention of the printing press was to literature (BENJAMIN, 1983).

Since its inception, photography has been used by police organisations as a means of surveillance and identification. However, problems made the image a less than convincing means in this process, such as the resistance of criminals to being photographed - often distorting expressions - the lack of standards in the photographic act and the lack of methodological archiving of images that would allow them to be used efficiently to recognise repeat offenders (GUNNING, 2004). In 1879, Alphonse Bertillon, a criminologist who began studies into anthropometric characterisation and classification in France, proposed standards and guidelines that would regulate photographic taking. He also proposed a new anthropometric identification method based on images, which he called signalling, also known as bertillonage. The method consisted of photographically recording the individual's face (from the front and in profile), marking and classifying common morphological characteristics, and cross-referencing this data so that previous images could be found without having to search through large quantities of images. The major problem with this identification system was its inability to provide uniformity in classifications, which is fundamental to underpinning the technical and scientific rigour needed in forensic sciences, where examinations are routinely carried out by different police officers (WILKINSON, 2008).

The main reason for applying facial studies in forensic science is the individuality of the human face. No two individuals have the same physical facial characteristics (GOLDSTEIN; HARMON; LESK, 1971). Even univitelline twins have facial differences that are perceptible to a lesser or greater degree, allowing each face to be related to a different individual (MACHADO et al., 2014). In principle, any method that records this individuality can be used in human identification processes.

Although the term recognition is defined as a method of empirical identification, while the term identification is defined as a method of scientific recognition, the term facial recognition, for the purposes of forensics, can refer to an empirical or scientific method. Empirical facial recognition can be seen, for example, in the facial comparison of individuals recorded in the memory of a witness or family member with the visualised image of a criminal or a victim; in the presumption of the visual appearance of a missing person, suspect of a crime or victim, in the so-called "false portrait"; and in the facial recognition provided by forensic facial reconstruction techniques (HENNEBERG; SIMPSON; STEPHAN, 2003).

As a scientific method, on the other hand, there is a linguistic contradiction due to the generic use of the expression recognition (a term known in forensic circles as the non-scientific determination of an individual's identity, therefore consisting of a subjective method). When this is carried out by means of a systematic comparison between facial images - a process known as facial mapping - the method is defined as 'Facial *Identification'* or *'Forensic Facial Analysis*', although the term '*Facial Recognition*' is universally used to refer to both empirical and scientific methods (GERRARD et al., 2007; LEE et al., 2009; STAVRIANOS et al., 2012).

The term "Face Recognition" is mainly used to refer to automated methods of recognising patterns and is one of the areas of study in biometric sciences, as are the studies of fingerprints, voice, retina, iris and hand geometry (MACHADO et al., 2014). It is one of the most discussed subjects in the field of computer science, which is actively seeking to develop algorithms capable of automating the comparative process of facial biometrics (REN; DAI, 2010; SAMAL; IYENGAR, 1992; SHI; SAMAI; MARX, 2006). From the beginning of its development in the second half of the 20th century to the present day, biometrics has gained a lot of prominence, especially in recent years, as it presents itself as an interesting alternative to traditional authentication systems such as passwords, PINs and smart cards (HOFER; MARANA, 2007).

The first attempts to automate facial identification began in the 1960s and, over time, systems have been developed and applied for commercial purposes, law enforcement, military purposes, airport security, access control to facilities, surveillance and monitoring, among others (HESS, 2010; LI et al., 2012). Facial comparison systems basically consist of one-to-one primary verification systems, in real time, where the system verifies that the person is who they say they are, and also identification systems, where one is compared to several, the latter being widely used in the facial identification process (LI et al., 2012).

Facial images can be used by anthropologists and forensic artists to progress the age of missing persons, with recreated images being a more faithful source of recognition than the images initially obtained. Notwithstanding the gathering of data for facial recognition to be established, these processes are extremely important, as they help and direct the determination of a person's identity through facial structures. Facial identification tests are also used in document fraud situations (PORTER; DORAN, 2000) and in the identification of rapists and paedophiles (TAYLOR et al., 1993), as they usually record their victims and themselves on videos and photographs.

Whenever images or videos are available at a crime scene, they can be used as an important tool for the investigation of the case by forensic scientists. Multimedia traces, as they are perennial records of a past reality, are important means of proof (BULUT; SEVIM, 2013; MACHADO et al., 2014) and are becoming increasingly common in Brazilian and global police cases. These traces can be produced by the investigation team itself, by the victim and/or the accused, on purpose, by chance, or even in a timely manner, such as those collected on so-called Closed (or Internal) Television Circuits (CCTV). These systems, usually installed in buildings and homes, have been an important tool in identifying and apprehending people involved in various crimes and in combating and preventing crime in general (GILL; SPRIGGS, 2005; GOOLD, 2002).

Although there is no official data, it is estimated that England has at least five million cameras distributed over its 130,400 km of land[2], making it the country with the highest density of internal circuit cameras in the world (DAVIS; VALENTINE; WILKINSON, 2012; McCAHILL; NORRIS, 2003; NORRIS; McCAHILL; WOOD, 2004). In the United States, in 2009 alone, it was estimated that more than 30 million security cameras were installed, resulting in a possible four billion hours of filming per week (VLAHOS, 2009). This large-scale implementation therefore seems inevitable in every country in the world (DAVIS; VALENTINE; WILKINSON, 2012; NORRIS; McCAHILL; WOOD, 2004). In the field of Criminal Forensics, there are more and more requests for tests to identify robbers of bank branches, lottery shops, ATMs, public institutions, private companies and condominiums, caught by these security systems committing such offences.

In contrast to this exponential growth in the production of images, there are several sources available for comparison, such as images acquired from passports, identity cards, traffic licences and criminal records routinely taken by judicial and forensic bodies around the world (KRISHAN; KANCHAN, 2012). In the United States, these photographic records are referred to as "mug shots" and are characterised by two facial photographs, one frontal and the other in profile (PORTER; DORAN, 2000). This factor greatly contributes to the applicability and viability of facial identification processes, since their determination depends on comparative systems.

Although security cameras and other video recording devices are capable of capturing reliable three-dimensional images, the comparison of facial images will generally fall back on two-dimensional images (HENNEBERG; SIMPSON; STEPHAN, 2003; MORECROFT; FIELLER; EVISON, 2010). Facial identification systems carried out on images are largely influenced by variations in lighting conditions, viewing direction or poses, facial expressions, ageing, the use of adornments and disguises and the time elapsed between obtaining the images, sources of comparison (DAVIS; VALENTINE; WILKINSON, 2012; LEE, 2009; LI et al., 2012). Factors related to the image recording equipment can also significantly influence the accuracy of facial identification, such as the focal length of the lens, which can affect the proportion and shape of some features (EDMOND et al., 2009; HARPER; LATTO, 2001), the use of lenses such as wide-angle lenses (used in cash machines to widen the viewing angle) and telephoto lenses (used to zoom in on images), which can produce distortions (DAVIS; VALENTINE; WILKINSON, 2012).

The Facial *Identification Scientific Working Group* (FISWG) was set up to gather and disseminate accurate information on the correct application of methodologies and technologies for facial identification and automated facial recognition systems. The FISWG aims to develop standards, guidelines and best practices in image-based facial comparisons, as well as providing recommendations that contribute to the advancement of research and development in this scientific field. The FISWG documents differentiate between *facial examination* and facial review (FISWIG, 2012). Both are defined as facial comparison procedures, but facial examination is carried out by specialised professionals using rigorous methods and procedures as an identification process. According to the FISWG (2012), facial identification can be carried out using four different methods:

a) Holistic: These are methods based on the natural human ability to classify and recognise faces, taking into account all the features viewed simultaneously. These methods are not recommended for forensic purposes, as they bring with them a high degree of subjectivity, incompatible with the neutrality that forensic examination requires. They should only be used when time is restricted (FISWG, 2012; MACHADO et al., 2014).

b) Morphological: These are methods in which facial anatomical features are identified and classified into different categories (as attributes of similarity or divergence) and in relation to their discriminatory capacity. Despite their great subjectivity, these methods are considered the main ones for carrying out facial comparison examinations for forensic purposes by the FISWG, especially in images with low resolution, taken at different angles, or when individualising characteristics are clearly present (DAVIS; VALENTINE; DAVIS, 2010; HENNEBERG; SIMPSON; STEPHAN, 2003). On the other hand, difficulties in these methods are observed when facial features have elements from more than one classification, when they are on the borderline of two classifications, or when they do not fit into any classification (DAVIS; VALENTINE; DAVIS, 2010). The discriminating power of faces with similar characteristics is extremely problematic (DAVIS; VALENTINE; DAVIS, 2010). In this sense, a single reliable difference is more valuable than several similar characteristics (DAVIS; VALENTINE; DAVIS, 2010). This technique is extremely dependent on the practice and experience of the examiners (KRISHAN; KANCHAN, 2012). According to FISWG recommendations, Brazilian forensic practice is based on this method for facial identification by images and suggests that, whenever the material allows, a complementary analysis by superimposition should be carried out (FISWG, 2012; MACHADO et al., 2014).

c) Photoanthropometric: These are methods used to analyse measurements and angles between cephalometric points on the compared faces (DAVIS; VALENTINE; DAVIS, 2010; FISWG, 2012; MACHADO et al., 2014). Accurate values can be obtained using this method, allowing for reliable assessment and parametric analyses (DAVIS; VALENTINE; DAVIS, 2010). However, problems are encountered when images are not aligned or when facial expressions are present. In these cases, a combination of photoanthropometric and morphological techniques can be useful for examining these images (DAVIS; VALENTINE; DAVIS, 2010; ROELOFSE; STEYN; BECKER, 2008). However, studies have shown that this method should not be used in forensic image examinations, either individually or in conjunction with other methods - mainly due to the gap in systematic comparison studies and the uncertainty caused even in ideal situations - nor in uncontrolled conditions (KLEINBERG et al., 2007; MORETON; MORLEY, 2011).

d) By superimposition: These are methods that create compositions between the questioned face and the so-called standard or known face, properly aligned and projected onto each other, in order to help visualise the differences and similarities of facial features, as well as the presence or absence of facial asymmetry (DAVIS; VALENTINE; DAVIS, 2010). Fading mechanisms can be used, where one image superimposed on the other is slowly made to disappear, highlighting the second image (Í§CAN, 1993), or visual oscillation mechanisms, where a vertical, horizontal or diagonal line erases one of the images at the same time as the other is revealed (DAVIS; VALENTINE; WILKINSON. 2012). They can only be used for forensic purposes in conjunction with morphological methods (FISWG, 2012; MACHADO et al., 2014). Research has been carried out analysing the techniques described and the difficulties associated with their application in forensic contexts. However, no method provides certainty of identification (DAVIS; VALENTINE; DAVIS, 2010). Despite this, this type of expert evidence has been accepted in courts in India, Italy, South Africa, the United States, the United Kingdom and elsewhere (DELIBERTI; OLSON, 1991). It is estimated that in the UK alone, more than 500 expert reports are issued every year (DAVIS; VALENTINE; DAVIS, 2010). This makes it clear that it is important to specify equipment and related procedures for capturing images, as well as definitions and methodologies for facial comparison in images, the basic elements of which are based on their anatomical reference points. The absence of a scientific method in facial comparison is unacceptable from an expert point of view, and its use without the appropriate standards and related studies can lead to justice not being applied, its improper application or, even more seriously, unjust condemnation through erroneous application.

1.6. Photoanthropometry: The Image as a Source of Information

Photoanthropometry is a relatively recent science and arose from the need to establish methodologies for analysing anthropometric images. It is defined as the analysis of points, dimensions and anthropometric angles to quantify facial features and proportions in a photograph (Í§CAN, 1993). Its main objective is to obtain information about the real objects illustrated in the two-dimensional image and to metrically compare proportion relationships between one photograph and another, as opposed to the search for visual differences and similarities characteristic of morphological comparisons (DAVIS; VALENTINE; DAVIS, 2010; ÍÇCAN; LOTH, 2000; KAU et al., 2007; RAI; KAUR, 2013).

The traditional photoanthropometric approach involves identifying a number of anatomical points in the image and measuring the distances between them (ALLEN, 2008; MORETON; MORLEY, 2011). In order for proportions, indices and angles to be measured, instead of using linear measurements, these distances can be normalised by dividing them by the interpupillary distance, for example (KLEINBERG et al., 2007; PORTER; DORAN, 2000). The so-called Normalised Proportionality Indices (PIs) can be used in the photoanthropometric comparison of a questioned image with the reference image, and are calculated for each measurement as a percentage of it by the largest measurement available (KLEINBERG et al., 2007; MORETON; MORLEY, 2011). However, their use is not sufficiently discriminating to positively identify an individual (KLEINBERG et al., 2007) and they are currently indicated for exclusion tests (DAVIS; VALENTINE; DAVIS, 2010; MORETON; MORLEY, 2011).

Photoanthropometry can be carried out directly on images, using rulers and protractors, or mathematically, after digitising the image (BATTAGEL, 1993). When digitised, spatial coordinates are used for Euclidean Geometry calculations in order to obtain the same distances and angles as in conventional anthropometric methods (SFORZA et al., 2009). As these points are not determined directly and their definitions are not based on images, they may not have the same anatomical location as initially defined. Therefore, when possible, the analysis should be limited to only those that are clearly visualised (SFORZA et al., 2009). Measurements based on anatomical points in soft tissue, i.e. cephalometric points, may be more suitable for photoanthropometry, while for direct measurements, bony points that require palpation, such as craniometric points, would be preferable (DOUGLAS, 2004; DILIBERTI; OLSON, 1991).

One of the advantages of taking measurements from a photograph, as opposed to direct analysis, is that it does not require the individual's co-operation, consent or knowledge (DAVIS; VALENTINE; WILKINSON, 2012; RAS et al., 1996), nor does it require them to remain still for long periods of time. This aspect alone makes it difficult to apply direct examinations to children (FARKAS, 1996). In addition, taking photographs is generally quicker and requires less interaction with the examinee than when measurements are taken manually (DOUGLAS, 2004; DOUGLAS; MUTSVANGWA, 2010). If necessary, measurements from photographs can be repeated, whereas repeating direct measurements may not be possible (DOUGLAS; MUTSVANGWA, 2010). Unlike some measurements obtained directly, such as those taken around the eyes, measurements on images are painless and pose no risk to the examinee (DOUGLAS, 2004).

On the other hand, due to the absence of a description based on images, the reference points may be more evident and identifiable when analysed directly (Í§CAN, 1993), and, when possible, they should be marked directly on the face before the photograph is taken (DOUGLAS; MUTSVANGWA, 2010). Photographs need some measure of scale, otherwise only proportions of measurements can be compared (DOUGLAS; MUTSVANGWA, 2010). A common disadvantage that hinders and sometimes prevents the use of images for facial analysis purposes is the methodological sensitivity to variations in the environment, such as lighting, pose, expression and ageing (SHI; SAMAI; MARX, 2006). A good photoanthropometric measurement system must be able to extract as many dissimilarities as possible between different individuals and at the same time be independent of these variations.

Although automated analysis systems are on the rise, facial images are becoming increasingly important in biometrics and anthropological research (DEMAYO et al., 2009, HENNESSY; MOSS, 2001), as they are relatively cheap and accessible means of recording the bank of information that makes up the human face (MACHADO et al., 2014). The standardisation of facial examinations in images is necessary, given that definitions and structural references used in craniofacial anthropometry were originally developed for direct analyses and, depending on their anatomical position, become imperceptible in images, thus increasing the subjectivity of analyses, especially when determined by different examiners. In order to make examinations more accurate, it is essential to establish and standardise, initially, topographical and structural references that can only be seen in the images, a process that has not yet been carried out in international literature. The vast majority of studies on photoanthropometric analysis assess the reliability of photoanthropometric measurements by comparing them with direct measurements, without, however, worrying about transferring the definitions of anatomical reference points to applications in facial images.

Despite the wide area of application of photoanthropometry and its growing demand in the forensic sciences, studies warn of the difficulties associated with the method, especially when used for human identification. Currently, no method provides great certainty in this determination, which justifies the need for research that initially seeks to standardise the description of anatomical reference points so that they can be identified in frontal images, as well as standardising analysis methodologies so that there can be a comparison and, consequently, progression of studies in this area. In this context, great care must be taken to present this evidence in court in order to obtain a conviction that is not based on alternative evidence (DAVIS; VALENTINE; WILKINSON, 2012).

1.6.1. Limitations of the Methods

Studies have shown that it is possible to easily identify a known person from the face obtained from images and videos, even when they are of poor quality. However, this task becomes arduous when we don't know the person (BRUCE et al., 2001; BURTON et al., 1999; DAVIS; VALENTINE; DAVIS, 2010). The performance of automated facial identification systems is superior to human perception under normal ideal conditions. However, accuracy is severely impaired in non-ideal conditions, a fact that corroborates the difficulty of their acceptance by law enforcement agencies in forensic cases (BURTON et al., 2001; PHILLIPS; SCRUGGS; O'TOOLE, 2007).

Digital CCTV systems require high processing, storage and data transmission capacity, which of course comes at a relatively high cost (KEVAL; SASSE, 2008). Many owners of these systems end up compromising on the quality of the video in order to reduce the costs of its implementation . Unfortunately, the production of potentially usable video for the main security observation tasks, such as monitoring, detection, recognition and identification, turns out to be tiny compared to the amount of images produced (ALDRIDGE, 1994).

It is estimated that 89 per cent of the CCTV images that reach the police are far from ideal. This rate was confirmed by the 2007 National CCTV Strategy (United States), which suggested that more than 80 per cent of the evidence provided to the police from CCTV is far from ideal. Currently, such evidence is admitted in court even when there are weaknesses due to poor image quality (CARROLL-MAYER; FAIRWEATHER; STAHL, 2008). Non-forensic and/or fully automated scenarios are not severely impacted by degradation and performance factors (JAIN; BRENDAN; UNSANG, 2012). However, a major demand for these analyses is precisely non-automated facial identification forensics. The literature on non-automated image comparison is scarce, and even the articles that do deal with the subject end up including extensive material on automated methods, mainly due to the strong academic aspect of the subject (ALI;

VELDHUIS; SPREEUWERS, 2010; MACHADO et al., 2014).

Unlike other identification methods, such as DNA and fingerprints, facial proportions are not fixed, absolute characteristics. Facial features are dynamic, changeable and easily altered by a myriad of different factors, whether physical (such as age, weight and the presence of injuries or illnesses) or extrinsic (such as lighting, the focal length of the camera or the angle of the head) (MORETON; MORLEY, 2011). If photoanthropometry is to be used in the courts, it is essential that the influence of extrinsic variables is investigated empirically (MORETON; MORLEY, 2011).

Generally speaking, the facial identification scientific community recognises four main factors that significantly compromise identification accuracy. These are pose, lighting, expression and ageing (JAIN; BRENDAN; UNSANG, 2012). Added to these factors are the low resolution of the images, the lack of contrast, the presence of different types of noise and disturbances, shaking caused by movement and/or lack of focus, geometric distortions that limit the reconstruction of the dimensions of the objects within the image and images with different angles (LEE et al., 2009).

In order to overcome these adversities, software and frameworks have been proposed to improve the reproducibility and reliability of these analyses. An example of this is the FI2 (Image Investigation Tool) software (HENRIQUES et al., 2012). Image pre-processing, defined as any process designed to improve its visual appearance (SWDIG, 2004), can and should be applied in order to reduce these image distortion factors (BULUT; SEVIM, 2013).

CHAPTER 2

Otjetívo

The primary objective of this study was to propose a methodology for standardising cephalometric points based exclusively on frontal photographic images, and the points were henceforth referred to as photoanthropometric points. The purpose of the proposed methodology, produced in the form of a manual, was to standardise facial analyses for possible application in human identification examinations. It also aimed to determine, based on the proposed analysis technique and the limits of the methodology adopted in this work, which photoanthropometric points showed the greatest and least variability in measurement in each of the phases and which points showed the greatest reduction in variability with the adoption of the proposed methodology.

CHAPTER 3

Materials and Methods

3.1. ***Ethical aspects***

Initially, the research project was submitted to the Research Ethics Committee of the Ribeirão Preto School of Dentistry at the University of São Paulo (CEP - FORP USP) and was approved under CAAE registration no. 17902713.7.0000.5419 (Annex A). The requests included the use of images of the research participants, acquired from an image bank, as well as the examiners responsible for the markings. A specific consent form for the use and dissemination of the reference images used in the proposed manual was obtained from the respective research participant.

3.2. ***General Study Design***

This study was based on analysing frontal images to verify the variability in the measurement of facial anatomical reference points. As these were originally established for direct determination on the human face, their definitions often do not allow them to be applied to images, leading to an increase in the variability of their measurement. The experimental part of the study was outlined in two stages, divided according to the description methodology used to mark the anatomical points. In the first phase, the conventional method (classic cephalometric) was used, and in the second, the photoanthropometric method proposed in this study, using references that can be visualised in frontal view facial images.

In both phases, 18 frontal facial images were used, randomly chosen from an image bank. Each image was analysed by five examiners with training and experience in craniofacial anatomy, three biomedical and two dental surgeons who carry out academic research in the area of craniofacial anatomy. Five photographs were analysed twice for intra-examiner analysis. For all the analyses, software developed by the Audiovisual and Electronic Forensics Service of the National Criminalistics Institute of the Federal Police, called SMVFace, was used, which was kindly provided for this study. Each examiner marked 16 facial points on each photograph. These points were chosen according to the feasibility of visualising them in frontal view and according to the routine literary presentation in studies related to photoanthropometry, specifically in the forensic area. With the exception of the Glabella point - a point on the neurocranium - only prosopometric points on the viscerocranium were considered as references, as they are less complex to determine due to the lack of anatomical overlap with other structures.

Measurements were made on the face and on the photograph of one of the research subjects in order to establish a conversion of the image pixels with the measurement in millimetres on the face. To do this, two examiners took three measurements of the Ectocanthion-Ectocanthion and Chelion-Chelion distances directly on the face and indirectly on the corresponding image, using the same software. Although the inter- and intra-examiner values were very close, if not coincidental, an average of the values was obtained, arriving at a correspondence of four image pixels for every millimetre of the face.

Statistical tests were used to check the variability of the point markings between the phases and in each phase separately. Tests were also carried out to measure each examiner's error, using the interpupillary distance of the reference photograph as a reference, and to analyse intra-examiner variability within each of the phases. The methodology is detailed below.

3.3. ***Material***

The SMVFace software was developed specifically to be a tool for analysing facial images, allowing anatomical landmarks made by several examiners to be included in a single database, obtaining a reading of their position using an (x,y) coordinate in pixels. The information collected was stored in real time, making it possible to tabulate and analyse the results in a standardised and automated way (Figure 1). For the analyses, the software was previously installed on the computers used by the examiners, with conventional operating systems installed.

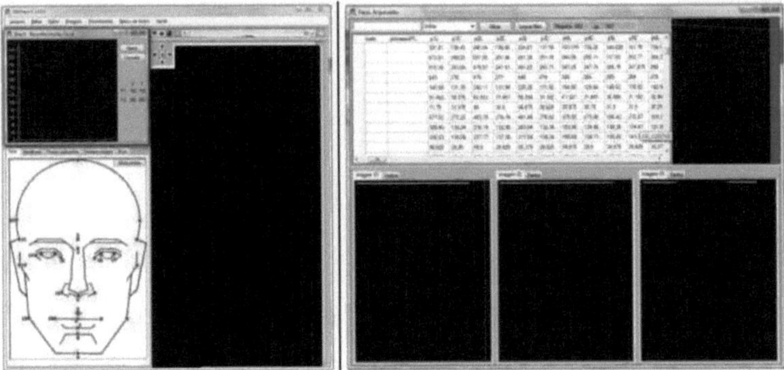

Figure 1. The image on the left shows the main interface of the programme used in the study. On the right, you can see the programme's database module, with the coordinates of each of the points marked by the examiners, already tabulated.

3.4. Method

3.4.1. Samples

3.4.1.1. Sample selection

The photographs used in all phases of this study were acquired from an image bank, kindly provided by those responsible for the project entitled "Genetics of the Face", carried out through a partnership between the Ribeirão Preto Medical School - USP, the University of Toronto (Canada) and the University of Sheffield (United Kingdom, England). The images were taken with the camera positioned at eye level at approximately 1.20 metres.

distance from the person being photographed, avoiding geometric distortion and ensuring adequate depth of field. All the photographs analysed were 1,200 pixels wide by 1,600 pixels high. The research subjects were orientated so that their eyes were directly facing the camera and the Frankfurt plane was positioned parallel to the ground. This plane is a standard horizontal reference for positioning the patient in photographs and cephalometric radiographs and is defined as a line that tangulates the upper edge of the external auditory canal and the lower edge of the infraorbital arch (ZIMBLER; HAM, 2005). The definition used in this study was drawn up by Zimbler and Ham, 2005, as the transition point between the lower eyelid and the skin of the cheek.

No optical zoom was used for the photographs.

To choose the images to be used, a double randomisation process was carried out, where 100 images (50 of males and 50 of females) were pre-selected from the 500 images initially in the database. These images were selected according to the exclusion and inclusion criteria presented in section 3.4.1.2. Of these images, 30 were chosen using the Excel programme®, where random numbers were generated for each image and, after numerical reorganisation, 10 images of males and 10 of females were chosen in ascending order of numbering. The sample was subsequently reduced to 18 images (nine male and nine female) due to the presence of reflections in the iris region which made it difficult to analyse the Medial Iridium and Lateral Iridium points.

3.3.1.1. Exclusion and inclusion criteria

Initially, the exclusion criterion was the failure to visualise the basic analysis structures for the study, due to the use of adornments, excessive cosmetic products, beards or moustaches, or the presence of hair covering the analysis regions. People with severe asymmetries and facial deformities were also excluded. Photographs with faces that suggested that the facial muscles were not relaxed, such as the presence of unusual expressions, smiling or partially open eyes, were also excluded from the analysis.

As inclusion criteria, the images were selected based on the following criteria:

1. Face centred in relation to the longitudinal axis. For this analysis, the reference adopted was symmetry in the visualisation of the two ears (pinna) (Figure 2).

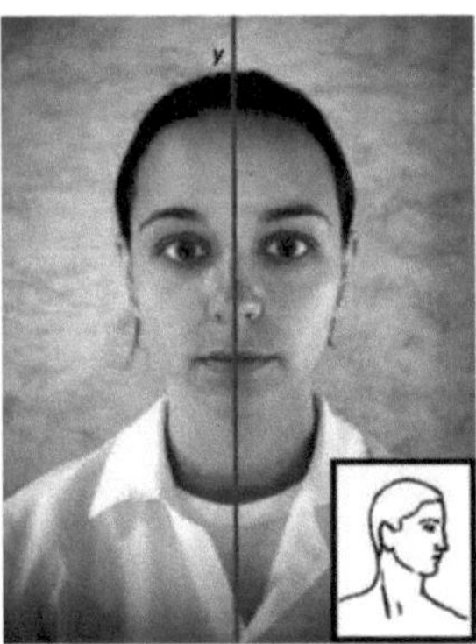

Figure 2 - Representation of the longitudinal axis (larger image) and changes in the position of the face (smaller image) when rotated in relation to this plane. Note that in extreme rotation in relation to this plane, one of the two pinnae is not visualised.

2. Face centred in relation to the transverse axis (laterolateral). For this analysis, the reference adopted was the alignment between the upper edge of the ear and the bipupillary line (Figure 3);

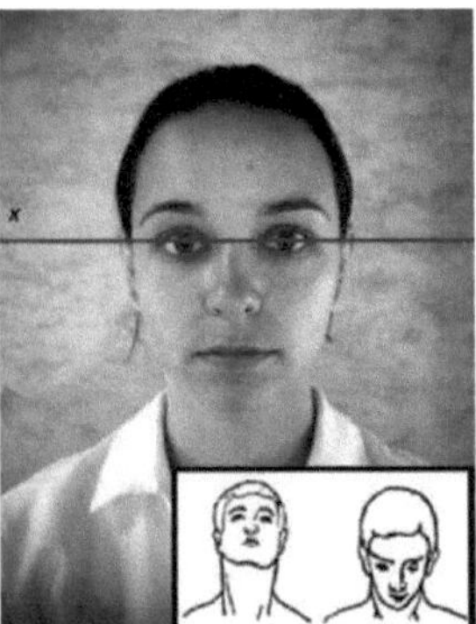

Figure 3: Representation of the transverse line (larger image) and changes in the positioning of the face (smaller image) when rotated in relation to this plane. Note that with the change in positioning in relation to this axis, the bipupillary line no longer coincides with the upper edge of the pinnae.

2. Face centred in relation to the sagittal (anteroposterior) axis. For this analysis, the reference adopted was the alignment between the upper edge of the ear and the bipupillary line (Figure 4).

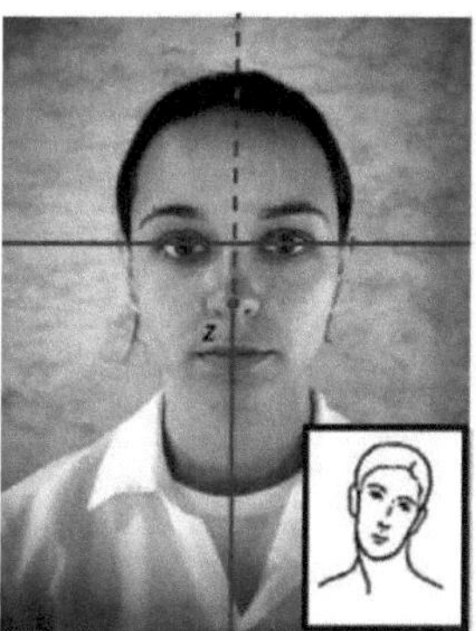

Figure 4 - Representation of the sagittal axis (larger image) and change in the position of the face (smaller image) when rotated in relation to this plane. Note that the bipupillary line is horizontal.

3.4.2. Experimental Phase

In both phases of the experimental study, each examiner analysed 18 frontal photographs of adult men and women. After explaining how to use the software, each of the five examiners was given a description of the anatomical references. In the first phase, they were given the cephalometric descriptions, while in the second phase they were given the photoanthropometric description proposed in this study, both described in sections 3.4.2.1. and 3.4.2.2. Based on these descriptions, the examiners were instructed to mark 16 cephalometric points, eight odd (median) and eight even (lateral), totalling 24 cephalometric points (Figure 5) on the facial topography of the photographic projections. The points used in this study are in line with the cephalometric reference points and anatomical soft tissue points used by the authors George (2007), Kolar and Salter (1997), Cattaneo et al. (2012) and Zimbler and Ham (2005) (Figure 5).

Five photographs were analysed twice by the same researchers in each phase in order to check intra-observer variability, making a total of 23 analyses. In both phases, five faces were previously marked, strictly following the methodological description that would be used next, so that any doubts or difficulties regarding the use of the software could be resolved.

The analyses were carried out one day apart. On the first day, 18 photographs were analysed, divided between the morning, afternoon and evening, with two-hour intervals between each shift and a 15-minute rest after each hour of analysis. On the second day, five of the 18 photographs analysed the previous day were analysed in order to check intra-examiner variability. On the third and fourth days, the analyses were carried out in the same way, with the only difference being the description used. The order in which the faces were marked, as well as their numbering in each stage, was different due to prior randomisation using the Excel programme® . The descriptions were printed out and given to the examiners **(Table 2 and Appendix A)**, as was the order in which they were to be examined. The different experimental phases and their characteristics are summarised in **Table 1**.

Table 1. Summary of the experimental study according to the analysis phase and its characteristics.

Experimental Phase	**Phase 1**	**Phase 2**
Examiners	5	5
Photographs analysed	18	18
Photographs analysed twice	5	5
Points analysed	24	24
Description technique adopted	Cephalometric	Photoanthropometry

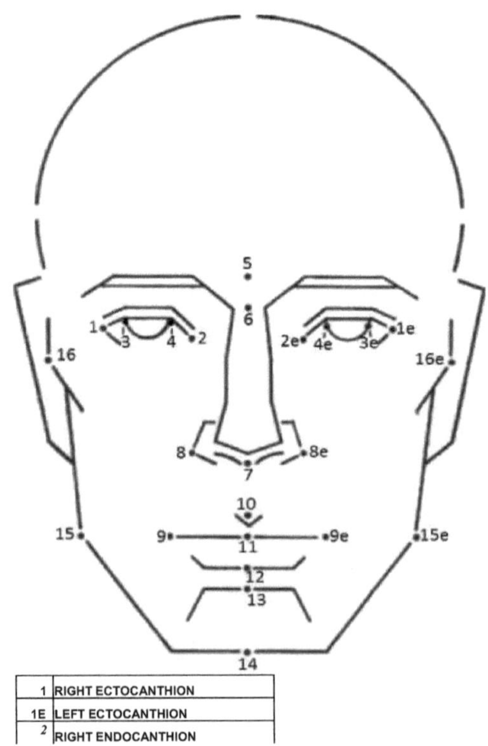

2E	LEFT ENDOCANTHION
3	IRIDIO RIGHT SIDE
3E	LEFT-BACK IRIDIUM
	RIGHT MEDIAL IRIDIUM
4E	LEFT MIDDLE IRON
&	GLABELLA
i	NÁSIO
7	SU8NASAL
B	ALAR RIGHT
BE	LEFT ALAR
4	RIGHT CHELION
BE	LEFT CHELION
1t>	UPPER LIP
11	STOMACH
12	LOWER LIP
13	LABIOMENTAL
14	GNÁT1O
1$	RIGHT GENIUS
16E	LEFT GENIUS
i£	RIGHT ZIGGER
1SE	ZIGIO LEFT

Figure 5: Location of the 24 (twenty-four) reference points that were adopted.

3.4.2.I. Facial Analysis Methodology - Phase 1

The descriptions of the anatomical landmarks used in this phase were those commonly found in the literature and are listed in **Table 2**.

Table 2: Anatomical description of the cephalometric points given to the examiners according to the authors George (2007), Kolar and Salter (1997), Cattaneo et al. (2012) and Zimbler and Ham (2005) (First Phase).

POINTS	DESCRIPTION
1. ectocanthion (ex)	Lateral angle of the eye.
2. Endocanthion	Medial angle of the eye. Medial corner of the eye where the eyelids meet, not the caruncles (reddish eminence in the medial region of the eye).
3. Lateral Iridium (il)	Lateral point of the iris (right or left eye).
4. Medial Iridium (im)	Medial point of the iris (right or left eye).
5. Glabella (g)	Most prominent region in the median sagittal plane between the supraorbital arches.
6. Násio (n)	Median point on the nasal root (apex of the frontonasal angle).
7. Subnasal (sn)	Midpoint of the base of the columella, below the nasal spine.
8. Alar (al)	Lateral point of the wing of the nose. Most lateral and posterior point of the curvature of the base of the nasal ala.
9. Chelion (ch)	Area where the white line of the upper and lower lip meets.
10. Upper lip (Is)	Midpoint on the white line of the upper lip.
11. Stomium (sto)	Meeting of the upper and lower lip in the median plane.
12. Lower lip (li)	Midpoint on the white line of the lower lip.
13. Labiomental (Im)	Point of greatest depression between lower lip and chin.
14. Gnatio (gn)	Lowest point in the middle region of the lower edge of the chin.
15. Genius (go)	Lateral point of the jaw angle.
16. Zygium (zy)	Most lateral point (greatest width) of the zygomatic bone in frontal view.

3.4.2.2. Facial Analysis Methodology - Phase 2

In this phase of the study, the examiners were instructed to apply a systematised demarcation technique based on a previous descriptive explanation of the points (anatomical and operational) presented in Appendix A, in the form of a manual, the product of this master's thesis, drawn up in partnership with the Federal Police and in layman's terms for use in future studies with examiners with no knowledge of craniofacial anatomy. The description presented in this study was called a photoanthropometric description because it is based on anatomical structures that can be visually identified in frontal photographs.

To demarcate these points, tools and geometric figures (reference structures) available in the software were used to help visualise the points and guide the examiners' decisions on marking them. The mobile tools, such as the horizontal and vertical reference lines, could be removed and inserted into the analysis by the examiners at any time. The movable lines helped the examiners mark when descriptions such as "most lateral/median point" or "most inferior/superior point" were present. The fixed tools, on the other hand, appeared after the determination of pre-established points and required prior definitions, as well as the adjustment of the SMVFace software, so that they were automatically established during facial analyses. The definition of these fixed tools, as well as how they were set up, is described below.

> Orbital Midline: Fixed vertical reference line that appears on the image after determining the Endocanthion and Ectocanthion points of both hemifaces (right and left). This line was defined as the union of the two points formed by the intersection of two circles, both having the ectocanthion point of each facial side as their centre and the distance from this point to the Endocanthion point of the contralateral hemiface as their radius.

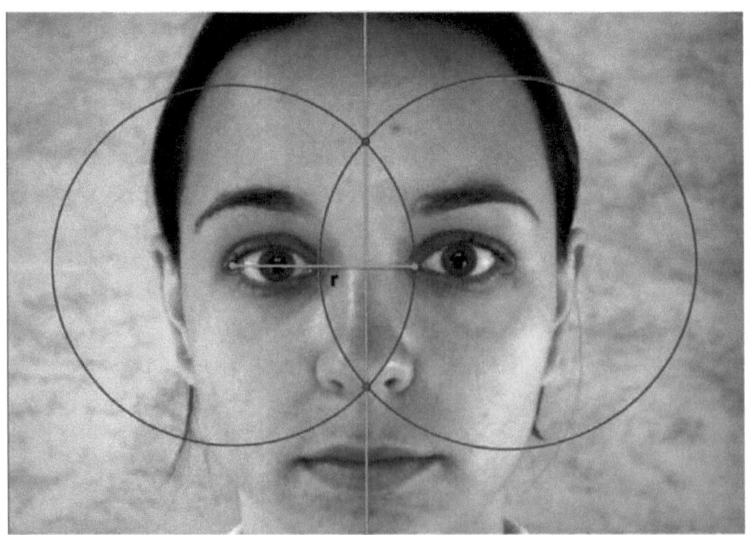

Figure 6 - Representation of how the orbital midline is obtained (green line). Two reference circles of each hemiface (shown in blue) are obtained, with the Ectocanthion points as centres and the Ectocanthion - contralateral Endocanthion distances (shown in orange) as radii (r). The intersection of the two circles (points in red) determines the orbital midline.

> Pupil Centre: Ocular reference point that appears after determining the four Iridium points (two for each hemiface), and is defined as the midpoint of the line drawn between the ipsilateral Lateral and Medial Iridiums. The pupil centres can vary in "y" (ordinate of the Cartesian coordinate plane) as a function of the variation in the position of their reference points (Iridions). An average in "y" of the lines representing these distances between the aforementioned ipsilateral points of each hemiface is defined automatically by the software to obtain the centre of the reference pupil (which has the same "y" position for both hemifaces).

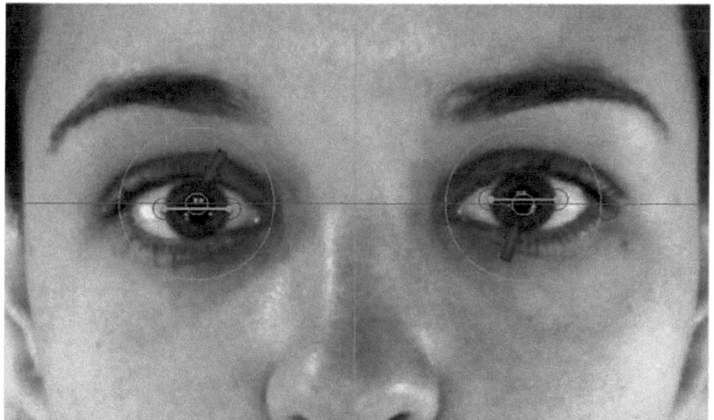

Figure 7. Representation of the pupil centres (red arrow). They are determined horizontally by the average of the distances between the ipsilateral Medial and Lateral Iridium points (lines in orange). Vertically, they are obtained by averaging the positions of the lines defined by these points. Note that the line representing the distance between the Medial and Lateral Iridions on the right is positioned below the same line on the left. The computer averages the two distances in "y" to determine the position of the pupil centres, which are on the same line and therefore in the same "y" position (shown in blue).

> Ocular Circumference: Circumference defined after determining the points Lateral Iridion and Medial Iridion of both hemifaces, determined as a circle with a pupil centre radius - Endocanthion. As the radii can be different on each hemiface, the average between the two values is calculated automatically by the software, determining the final radius of the

reference circumference.

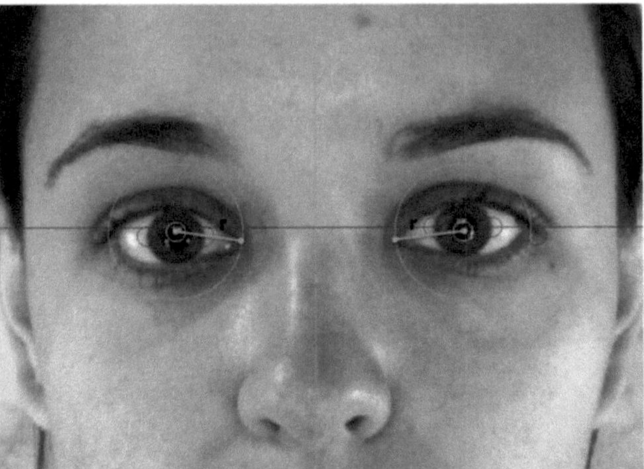

Figure 8. Representation of the ocular circumferences (grey lines). They are defined from the centre of the pupil and have as their radius (r) the distance pupil centre - ipsilateral Endocanthion (represented by the orange line). As these distances can be different for each hemiface, the final circumference will be defined by averaging the radii.

3.5. ***Statistical Analysis***

Once the data from the appointments made in Phases 1 and 2 of the study had been extracted from the SMVFace database, the information was tabulated and organised in Excel spreadsheet format®, for later forwarding to the statistics team. In order to simplify the study of the information and make it more didactic, the statistical analysis was segmented into five analysis groups, the objectives of which are summarised below:

1. Descriptive statistics
2. Assessment of normality
3. Analyses of variance
4. Analysingerror analysis
5. Intra-examinerintra-examiner

Two-dimensional coordinates of the 24 cephalometric points recorded in pixels were used as the source of information for the statistical analysis of the five analysis groups. This analysis was based on the coordinates of the points marked by the examiners on a non-visible Cartesian plane (x,y), with the lower left vertex of the images as the point of origin (x=0; y=0). The statistical analysis was based on three independent measurements:

1. Distance from the markings on the x-axis (Dx);

2. Distance from the markings on the y-axis (Dy);

3. Geometric distance observed between markings, also called "Euclidean distance" (De).

The independent analysis of "x" and "y" was adopted to make it possible to break down the variability and error of the markings, without which it would be impossible to understand the vectors associated with them. The third distance (De) was used to observe variability and error together. Graph 1 below illustrates the distances considered when analysing two hypothetical points (P1 and P2).

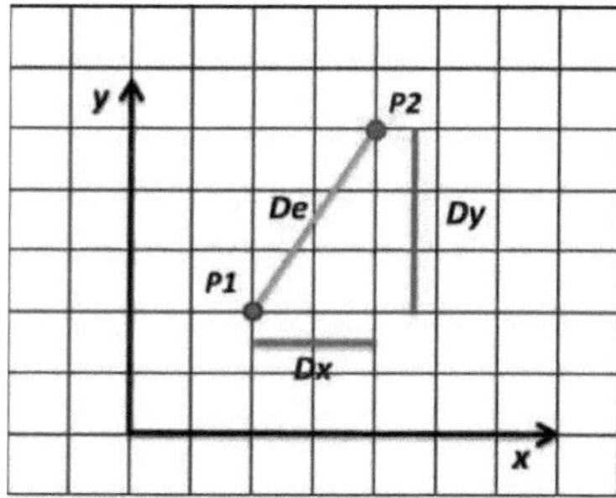

Graph 1: Representation of the reference distances used for statistical analyses between two hypothetical points, represented in blue (P1) and red (P2). Each square represents a pixel in the image. In the representation of the abscissa (x) and ordinate (y) on the Cartesian plane above, you can see: a green line, representing the Euclidean distance *(De);* a blue line, representing the distance in "x", corresponding to the abscissa (Dx); and a red line, representing the distance in "y", corresponding to the ordinate (Dy).

The information from the markings on the even (or bilateral) points was grouped together, given that the study did not aim to independently analyse the variance and error for the markings made on the left and right sides, but rather the differences between the non-homonymous points, considering the two different phases. Therefore, as the symmetrical homonymous points were considered as one, the results were presented for a total of 16 points, instead of the 24 points originally analysed (for example, the markings of the Right Chelion and Left Chelion points were grouped together and referred to only as Chelion). All the analyses described in this paper were carried out using the Microsoft Excel® 2013 computer programme and the SPSS version 14 statistics programme.

3.5.1. Descriptive Statistics

Descriptive statistics were used as the first stage of the analysis to provide general information on the distribution and behaviour of the data between Phases 1 and 2 (exploratory analysis), with special attention to measures of variability and dispersion, which will be discussed in a specific topic (Analysis of variance). Measures were taken of the mean, median, maximum, minimum, standard deviation, variance, coefficient of variation, among others, which guided the drawing up of specific graphs for each of the points in the two phases studied, considering the three measurements taken (Dx, Dy and De).

3.5.2. Assessment of normality

The Komolgorov-Smirnov test was used to assess the normality of the data, which was necessary for choosing the statistical methods adopted in the following stages of the study. The normality tests were carried out on the set of markings for each of the 16 points, in both phases, but considering the relative distances to the mean and not the absolute distance in pixels. This made it possible to group the relative measurements of different images in the same spreadsheet.

3.5.3. Analysis of variance

This group of analyses was carried out to detect differences in the variability of the marking of points between Phases 1 and 2 and between the markings of the same examiner within the same phase. At this stage, the relative distances between homonymous points were taken into account, as the variance was obtained in relation to the average of the markings. All the images were analysed together for each phase (n=90 for odd points and n=180 for even points, since there were 18 images analysed by five examiners). As the Komolgorov-Smirnof test indicated a normal distribution of the data, differences in variances were detected using the F test for homogeneity of variances, considering a significance level of 0.05 and a 95% confidence interval.

3.5.4. Error Analysis

Error analysis was used to see if the set of markings for the 16 points in each of the phases was within the acceptable standard error, using the interpupillary distance (IOD) as a reference. This way of analysing and evaluating the performance of the markings was based on the study by Çeliktutan, Ulukaya and Sankur (2013), who assumed that an error of up to 10% of the IOD was satisfactory, with the error given by the following formula:

$$\delta_i^k = \frac{d\{(x_i^k, y_i^k), (x_i^{\sim k}, y_i^{\sim k})\}}{\mathrm{IOD}},$$

Where d is the Euclidean distance calculated between the true coordinates (x, y) and the estimated coordinates (~x, ~y), normalised using the IOD. The superscript "k" indicates one of the anatomical points (e.g. Ectocanthion, Glabella, Nasion) and the subscript "i" is the image index. According to the study by Çeliktutan, Ulukaya and Sankur (2013), the error analysis in this study was carried out using acceptable errors of 10%, 5% and 1%, considering a 95% confidence interval.

3.5.5. Intra-examiner analysis

This group of analyses was carried out to check agreement in the markings of the same examiner, within the same phase, for the set of faces that were repeated (n=5 for each phase). Due to the small sample size, the non-parametric Wilcoxon test was used, with a significance level of 0.05 and a 95% confidence interval.

CHAPTER 4

Hediites

4.1. Descriptive statistics

The results of the descriptive analysis (mean, median, maximum, minimum, standard deviation and coefficient of variation) are presented in Appendix B. A summary of the average dispersion of the points, before and after the photoanthropometric description, is illustrated in Graph 1. This graph shows the variability of the Dx and Dy markings for each specific point, in both phases, in isolation and in relation to each other. It can be seen that some points show a great deal of initial variability (such as the Glabella, Nasion, Gonion, Zygium and Labiomental points), while others showed little variability in the first phase of the study (such as the Lateral Iridium, Medial Iridium, Subnasal and Lower Labial points, among others). It can also be seen that, for some points, the variation was predominant in some of the parameters analysed, such as greater variability in Dx (as in the Endocanthion, Ectocanthion and Chelion points in Phase 1) or greater variability in Dy (as in the Glabela, Násio, Gônio and Zígio points in Phase 1).

Analysing the variability of the markings between the phases, a topic that will be explored in greater depth in the "Analysis of Variance", it can be seen that, in general, there was a significant reduction in the variability of ***the*** marking of all the points. For some of them, the reduction was greater for the distance in "x" (as in the Endocanthion and Ectocanthion points, for example), while for others, the reduction was greater for the distance in "y" (as in the Glabela, Násio and Gônio points). The variation of both distances directly influences the variability of the Euclidean distance.

An exclusive analysis of the Euclidean distance, such as that carried out in the reference study by Çeliktutan, Ulukaya and Sankur (2013), results in the variability of the markings being visualised using the geometric figure of a circle, since the influence of the distances is not observed separately on the "x" (horizontal) and "y" (vertical) axes, unlike the isolated analysis of both distances (Dx and Dy) which are represented by an ellipse, as shown in Graph 2. Analysing Dx and Dy separately is extremely important when using indices, as greater variations on the "y" axis have a greater influence on the result for certain points, while for others, greater variations on the "x" axis are more significant. The study by Çeliktutan, Ulukaya and Sankur (2013) did not analyse the distances separately, probably because they were vector analyses, which are widely used for automated determination of anatomical reference points. For a better understanding of the variations, a detailed analysis of each phase will be presented below.

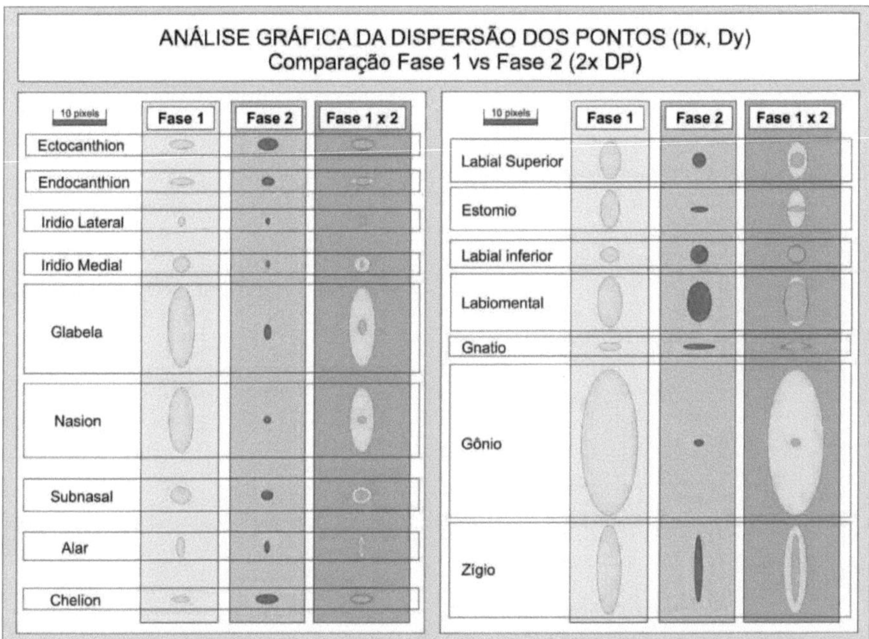

Graph 2: Graphical representation of the average dispersion (considering two standard deviations) of the markings obtained in both phases, for the "x" and "y" distances. The first column represents the average dispersion of Phase 1; the second, the average dispersion of Phase 2; the third column, the average dispersion of both superimposed. A scale of 10 pixels was used.

4.1.1. Phase One

Analysing the dispersion of the markings in each phase in isolation, and firstly the first phase, it can be seen that there was great variability in the determination of the Ionian cephalometric point in all three parameters analysed (Dx, Dy and De), with greater variability in Dy compared to Dx. The points with the greatest dispersion after the Ionian point were the Zygian, Glabella and Nasion points, in that order, for the Dy and De parameters. For the Dx parameter, the Glabela, Násio and Ectocanthion points were marked with the greatest variability, in this order **(Graph 3)**. As for the points with the lowest variability, the Lateral Iridium point was the one with the lowest variability in the two parameters analysed: Dx and De. For the Dy parameter, the Chelion point had the least variability, followed by the Endocanthion, Gnathion and Ectocanthion points **(Graph 4)**. The points with the least dispersion, considering the Euclidean distance, after the Lateral Iridium point, were the Chelion, Alar and Lower Labial points **(Graph 5)**. For Dx, the points with the least variability after the Lateral Iridium point were the Endocanthion, Gnathion and Ectocanthion points.

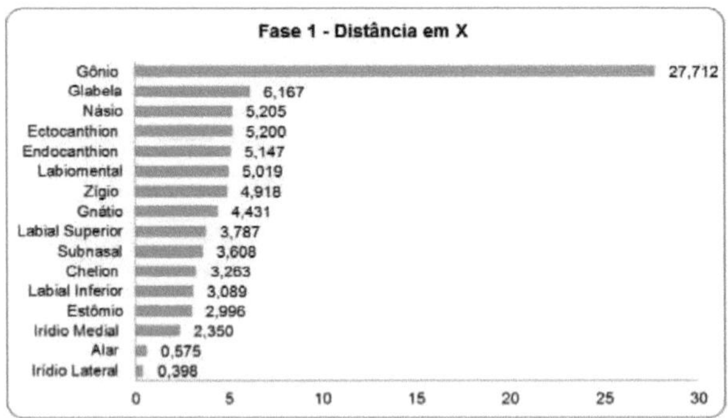

Graph 3: Result of the average dispersion per cephalometric point determined in the first phase, considering the distance in "x" (dispersion in pixels).

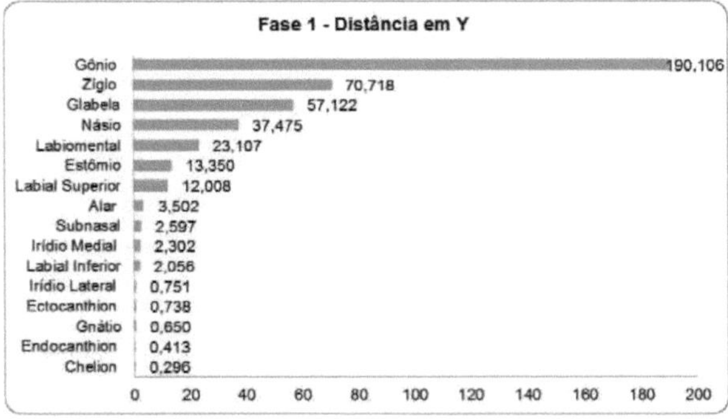

Graph 4: Result of the average dispersion per cephalometric point determined in the first phase, considering the distance in "y" (dispersion in pixels).

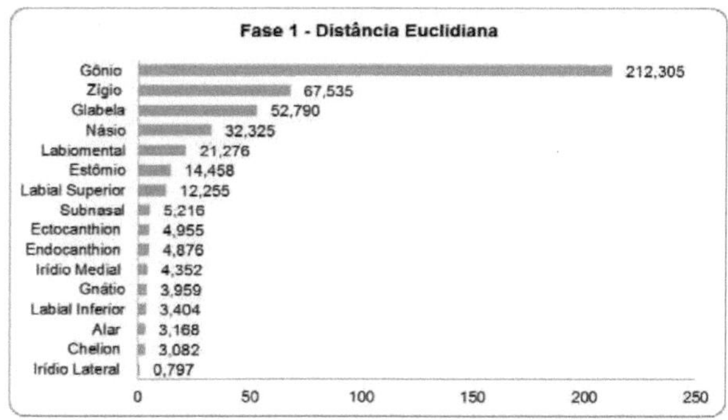

Graph 5: Result of the average dispersion per cephalometric point determined in the first phase, considering the Euclidean distance (dispersion in pixels).

4.1.2. Second Phase

As a result of the second phase, it can be seen that there was a significant reduction in the average variability of the markings in general**.** Analysing the dispersion shown only in Phase 2, it can be seen that the Gnatius point and the Zygion point showed the greatest dispersion, in Dx and in Dy and De, respectively. In Dx, the Labiomental, Chelion and Ectocanthion points showed the most variability after the Gnatius point **(Graph 6)**. For Dy, the Labiomental, Lower Labial and Glabella points; and for De, the Labiomental, Gnathion and Chelion points had the greatest dispersion in markings after the Zygian point. On the other hand, the Medial Iridium cephalometric point showed less dispersion in Dx, followed by the Lateral Iridium, Alar and Glabella points. In Dy, the Gnathius point showed the least dispersion, followed by the Stomium, Gonium and Lateral Iridium points **(Graph 7)**. The points with the lowest dispersion, considering the Euclidean distance, were Lateral Iridium, Medial Iridium, Nasium and Gonium, in that order **(Graph 8)**.

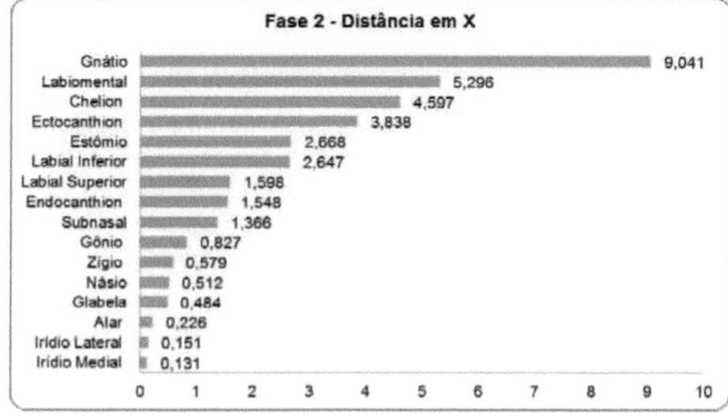

Graph 6: Result of the average dispersion per cephalometric point determined in the second phase, considering the distance in "x" (dispersion in pixels).

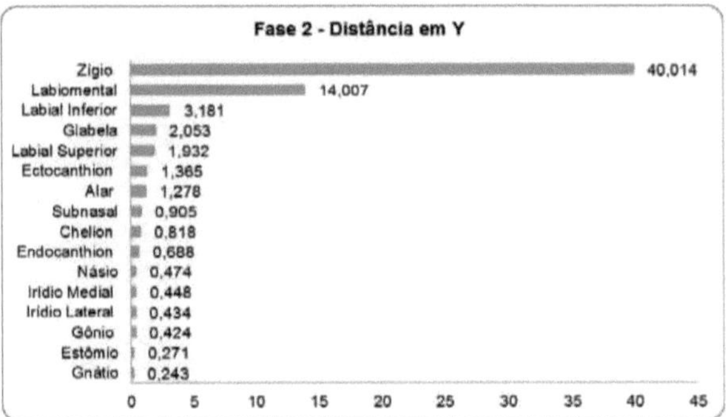

Graph 7: Result of the average dispersion per cephalometric point determined in the second phase, considering the distance in "y" (dispersion in pixels).

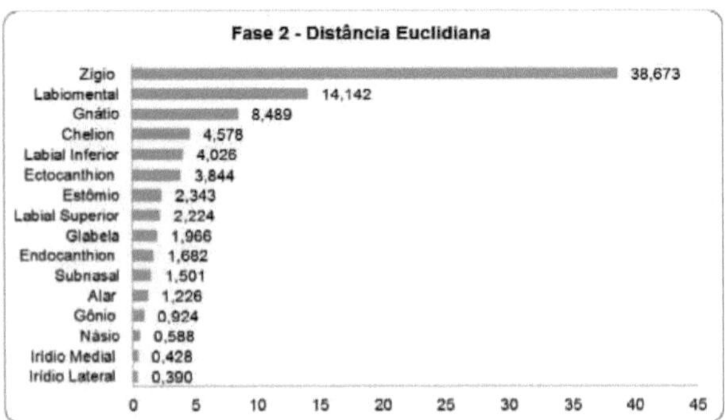

Graph 8: Result of the average dispersion per cephalometric point determined in the second phase, considering the Euclidean distance (dispersion in pixels).

4.2. *Assessment of normality*

The result of the Komolgorov-Smirnov test suggested that the study sample had a normal distribution, considering the assessment by relative distance, thus allowing homonymous points to be grouped together. This grouping resulted in the sample being multiplied by the number of images (18), totalling 90 samples for odd points and 180 for even points. Based on this observation, it was decided to use parametric tests to analyse variance and error. For the intra-examiner analysis, a non-parametric test was used, as described below.

4.3. *Analysis of variance*

Analysing the variability between the markings of the same examiner for each specific point, between the phases themselves and within the same phase, it can be seen that in Phase 1 the Gonius point showed great variability in marking, followed by the Zygian, Glabella, Nasion, Labiomental, Stomal, Labial Superior, Subnasal, Ectocanthion, Endocanthion, Medial Iridium, Gnathion, Labial Inferior, Alar, Chelion and Lateral Iridium points. In Phase 2, there was a reduction in variability in practically all the points, except for the Chelion, Gnathion and Labial Inferior points, which showed greater variability in Phase 2. Despite the increase in variability shown by these points, the application of the F test for homogeneity of variances showed that the variance of the Lower Labial point from Phase 1 to Phase 2 was the same, showing that there is no statistical evidence to affirm that the variation was different. This aspect was also observed in relation to the Ectocanthion point, showing a homogeneous reduction in variability and no statistical evidence of a difference. Analysing Phase 2, the point with the greatest measurement variability was the Zygian point, followed by the Labiomental, Gnathion, Chelion, Lower Labial, Ectocanthion, Stomal, Upper Labial, Glabella, Endocanthion, Subnasal, Alar, Gonium, Nasion, Medial Iridium and Lateral Iridium points. The order of the variance, by point and by phase, is shown in Table 3:

Table 3: Representation of the average variance in pixels, according to each phase and each specific point (Column: Variance). Presentation in ascending order of the variations (Column: Order) and classification of the variances according to the Phase being analysed (Column: *Ranking of the Phases)* where the number "1" represents the lowest variability and the number "2", the highest variability in the measurement of the anatomical reference points.

Location	Phase 1		Phase 2		Stage rankings	
	Variance	Order	Variance	Order	Phase 1	Phase 2
Alar	3,168	3	1,226	5	2	1
Chelion	3,082	2	4,578	13	1	2
Ectocanthion	4,955	8	3,844	11	2	1
Endocanthion	4,876	7	1,682	7	2	1
Stomach	14,458	11	2,343	10	2	1
Glabella	52,790	14	1,966	8	2	1
Gnatio	3,959	5	8,489	14	1	2
Ionian	212,305	16	0,924	4	2	1
Lateral Iridium	0,797	1	0,390	1	2	1
Medial Iridium	4,352	6	0,428	2	2	1
Lower lip	3,404	4	4,026	12	1	2
Upper lip	12,255	10	2,224	9	2	1
Labiomental	21,276	12	14,142	15	2	1
Násio	32,325	13	0,588	3	2	1
Subnasal	5,216	9	1,501	6	2	1
Zygian	67,535	15	38,673	16	2	1

By applying the hypothesis test and rejecting the null hypothesis at 5%, it can be seen that there was a highly significant reduction in the variation in the markings of the Alar, Endocanthion, Glabella, Gonion, Medial Iridium, Superior Labial and Zygian points when comparing Phase 1 with Phase 2 and in the three parameters analysed, obtaining a p-value of less than 0.0001. Not with such a high level of significance, but also significant, were the reductions in the variation of the markings of the Lateral Iridium, Nasion and Subnasal points, obtaining p-values of less than 0.001, 0.0041 and 0.0492, respectively. There was a significant reduction in the variations for all the analyses of the Stomal point, except for the "x" distance, where the variances were significantly the same, with a p-value of 0.2191.

For the Chelion point, a statistically significant increase in variation was observed in Phase 2 for all parameters, whereas what was expected was greater variation in Phase 1. For the Ectocanthion point, a significant reduction in variation was observed for the "x" distance parameter and for the Euclidean distance, which was curiously reversed when analysing the "y" distance, a fact that did not compromise the reduction in the point's variability.

Other points that deserve attention in this study were the Gnathion, Lower Labial and Labiomental points. The Gnatio point showed significantly different variations for all analyses, with p-values of <0.0003 for all parameters. However, the variations were significantly greater in Phase 2 for the "x" distance and Euclidean distance parameters. The Lower Labial point showed a reduction, but not significant for the distance in "x" (p-value <0.1516); an increase, but not significant, for the Euclidean distance parameter (p-value <0.1312); and a significant increase in variation for the distance in "y" parameter, obtaining a p-value of less than 0.0018 for this analysis. For the Labiomental point, there was a significant reduction (p-value <0.01) for the "y" distance parameter and a reduction, but not significant, for the Euclidean distance (p-value of 0.3598). There was a non-significant increase (p-value of

0.3598) in the variation for the "x" distance parameter.

4.4. ***Error analysis***

The following spreadsheets and graphs show the analysis of the Error in marking each specific point based on the "acceptable error" and the percentage of the Interpupillary Distance (IOD). As the IODs of each image showed little numerical variation between the 18 faces analysed, an average of these distances was taken to calculate the error, corresponding to a value of 261 pixels. In this study, 100% of the markings had errors of less than 5% of the IOD, which is why the analysis was based only on the error limit of 1% of the IOD. Calculating the value in pixels of the error limit considered in this study (1%), we obtain a value of 2.61 pixels for images with a resolution of 1200x1600, 3x4 aspect ratio.

4.4.1. Alar

As a result of analysing the error for the Alar point, it was possible to see that 86.67% of the markings made in Phase 2 (the percentage obtained from the difference between the total percentage and the percentage above the error for De, which in this case was 13.33%) were below the error of 1% of the interpupillary distance of the images, compared to 55.56% of the markings made in Phase 1, showing an error 70% lower than that observed for the same point in Phase 1.

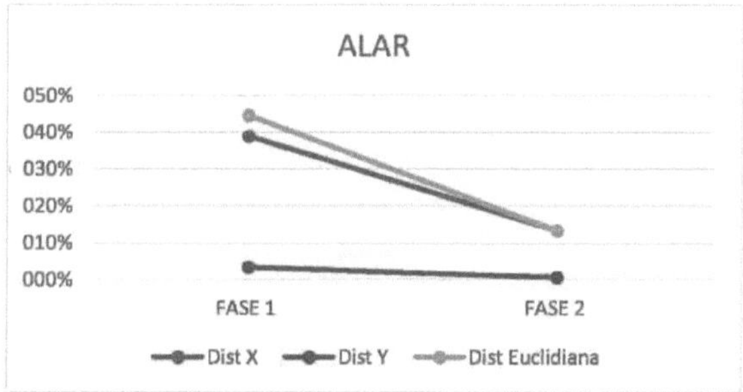

Graph 9: Percentage of markings above the 1% IOD error for the Alar point for the three parameters analysed (Scale 0-50%).

Table 4: Table referring to the previous graph showing the percentage of markings above the 1% IOD error for the Alar point for the three parameters analysed. The far right column shows the ratio of the error obtained in Phase 1 to Phase 2, in percentage, quantifying the reduction (-) or increase (+) in the error when comparing the two.

Alar	**Phase 1**	**Phase 2**	**Ratio (%)**
Dx	38,89%	13,33%	-65,71%
Dy	3,33%	0,56%	-83,33%
From	44,44%	13,33%	-70,00%

4.4.2. Chelion

Analysing the graph and table below, we can see an increase of 17.83% in the error of the markings in Phase 2 compared to Phase 1, as a result of the increase in variability between the phases. Despite the increase in variability and error in Phase 2, 56.67% of the markings were below 1% error in this phase.

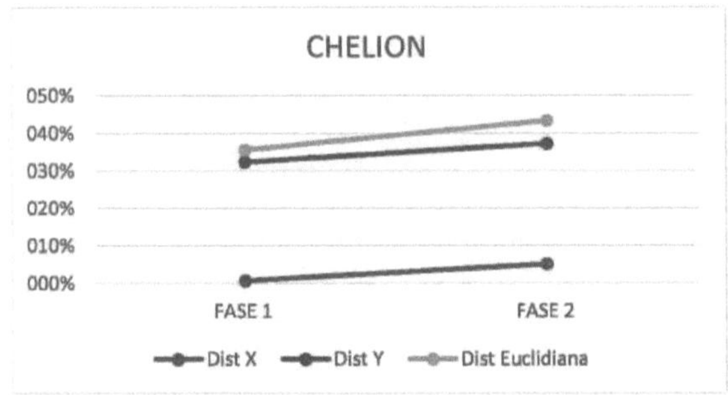

Graph 10: Percentage of markings above the 1% IOD error for the Chelion point for the three parameters analysed (Scale 0-50%).

Table 5: Table referring to the previous graph showing the percentage of markings above the 1% IOD error for the Chelion point for the three parameters analysed. The far right column shows the ratio of the error obtained in Phase 1 to Phase 2, in percentage, quantifying the reduction (-) or increase (+) in the error when comparing the two.

Chelion	Phase 1	Phase 2	Ratio (%)
Dx	0,56%	5,00%	+88,80%
Dy	32,22%	37,22%	+13,43%
From	35,56%	43,33%	+17,93%

4.4.3. Ectocanthion

For the Ectocanthion point, there was a 30.16 per cent reduction in marking error, with the percentage of markings above the 1 per cent error dropping from 70 per cent to 48.89 per cent.

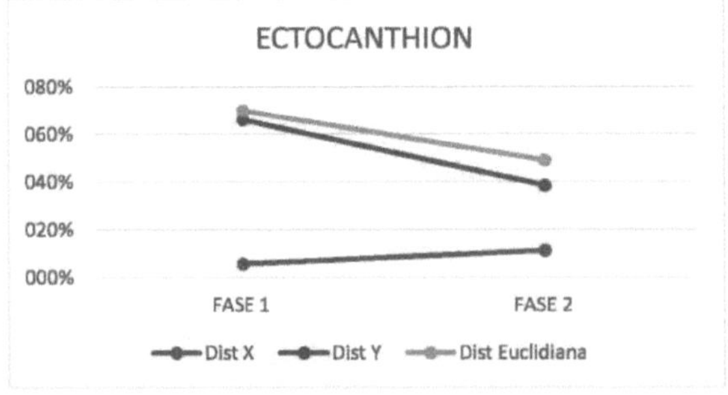

Graph 11: Percentage of markings above the 1% IOD error for the Ectocanthion point for the three parameters analysed (Scale 0-80%).

Table 6: Table referring to the previous graph showing the percentage of markings above the 1% IOD error for the Ectocanthion point for the three parameters analysed. The far right column shows the relationship between the error obtained in Phase 1 and Phase 2, in percentage, quantifying the reduction (-) or increase (+) in the error when comparing the two.

Ectocanthion	Phase 1	Phase 2	Ratio (%)
Dx	5,56%	11,11%	+49,95%
Dy	66,11%	38,33%	-42,02%

From	70,00%	48,89%	-30,16%

4.4.4. Endocanthion

It can be seen for the Endocanthion point that 82.22% of the markings, considering only the Phase 2 results, were below the 1% error of the interpupillary distance of the images, compared to 74.44% of the markings in Phase 1, showing a 30.44% reduction in marking error when comparing both phases. Despite the total reduction in error, there was an increase in error for Dx, restricting the percentage reduction in total error.

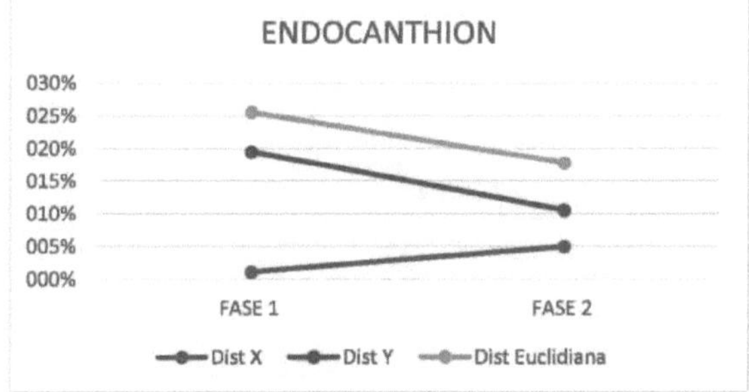

Graph 12: Percentage of markings above the 1% IOD error for the Endocanthion point for the three parameters analysed (Scale 0-30%).

Table 7: Table referring to the previous graph indicating the percentage of markings above the 1% error of the IOD referring to the Endocanthion point for the three parameters analysed. The far right column shows the relationship between the error obtained in Phase 1 and Phase 2, in percentage, quantifying the reduction (-) or increase (+) in the error when comparing the two.

Endocanthion	**Phase 1**	**Phase 2**	**Ratio (%)**
Dx	1,11%	5,00%	+77,80%
Dy	19,44%	10,56%	-45,68%
From	25,56%	17,78%	-30,44%

4.4.5. Glabella

Analysing the graph and table below, it can be seen that 74.44% of the Glabella point markings made in Phase 2 were below the 1% error of the interpupillary distance of the images, compared to just 2.22% of the markings made in Phase 1, showing a 73.86% reduction in error after using the photoanthropometric description.

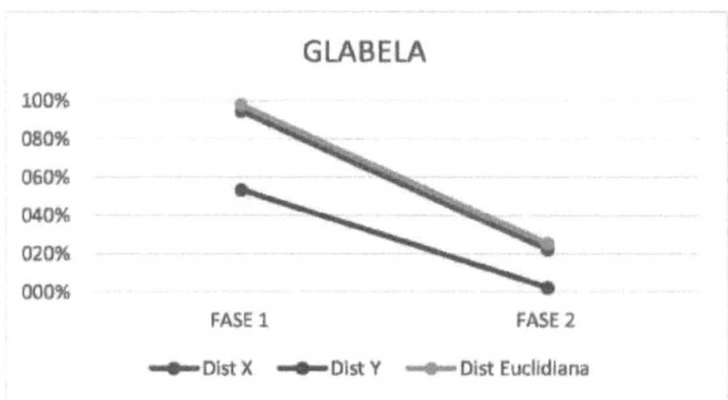

Graph 13: Percentage of markings above the 1% IOD error for the Glabela point for the three parameters analysed (Scale 0-100%).

Table 8: Table referring to the previous graph showing the percentage of markings above the 1% IOD error for the Glabela point for the three parameters analysed. The far right column shows the relationship between the error obtained in Phase 1 and Phase 2, in percentage, quantifying the reduction (-) or increase (+) in the error when comparing the two.

Glabella	**Phase 1**	**Phase 2**	**Ratio (%)**
Dx	94,44%	22,22%	-76,47%
Dy	53,33%	2,22%	-95,84%
From	97,78%	25,56%	-73,86%

4.4.6. Gnatio

For the Gnatio point, 57.78% of the markings made in Phase 2 were below the 1% error of the interpupillary distance of the images, compared to 51.78% of the markings in Phase 1, showing a 13.64% reduction in the error of the markings when comparing both phases.

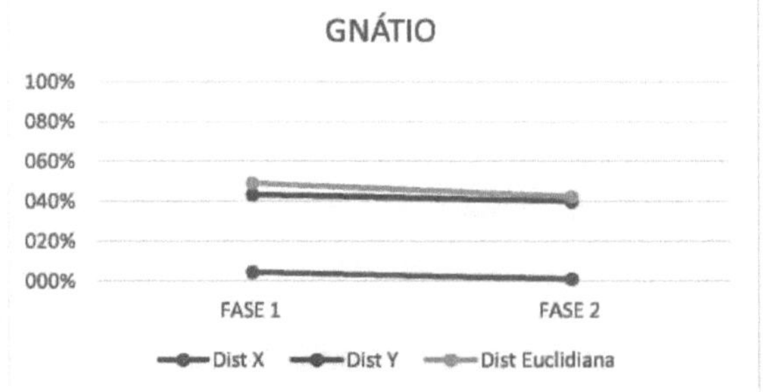

Graph 14: Percentage of markings above the 1% IOD error for the Gnatio point for the three parameters analysed (Scale 0-100%).

Table 9: Table referring to the previous graph showing the percentage of markings above the 1% IOD error for the Gnatio point for the three parameters analysed. The far right column shows the relationship between the error obtained in Phase 1 and Phase 2, in percentage, quantifying the reduction (-) or increase (+) in the error when comparing the two.

Gnatio	Phase 1	Phase 2	Ratio (%)
Dx	4,44%	1,11%	-75,00%
Dy	43,33%	40,00%	-7,69%
From	48,89%	42,22%	-13,64%

4.4.7. Ionium

Analysing the graph and table below, we can see that there was a 90.12% reduction in the error of the Ionian point markings after using the photoanthropometric description. Analysing Phase 2, 90.56% of the markings were below the 1% error of the interpupillary distance of the images, compared to 4.44% of the markings made in Phase 1.

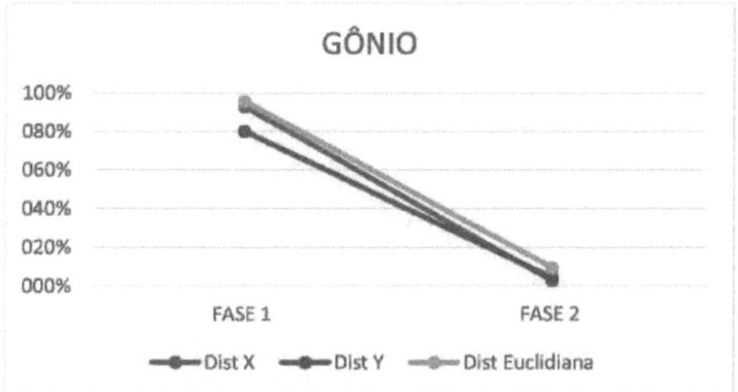

Graph 15: Percentage of markings above the 1% IOD error for the Gonio point for the three parameters analysed (Scale 0-100%).

Table 10: Table referring to the previous graph showing the percentage of markings above the 1% IOD error for the Gonio point for the three parameters analysed. The far right column shows the relationship between the error obtained in Phase 1 and Phase 2, in percentage, quantifying the reduction (-) or increase (+) in the error when comparing the two.

Ionian	Phase 1	Phase 2	Ratio (%)
Dx	92,99%	2,78%	-97,01%
Dy	80,00%	4,44%	-94,45%
From	95,56%	9,44%	-90,12%

4.4.8. Lateral Iridium

Although the initial error observed for the Lateral Iridium point in Phase 1 was small (only 11.67% of the markings were made above the IOD error of 1%), it can be seen that there was a reduction of 80.98% after using the photoanthropometric description, resulting in an error rate of 2.22% in Phase 2.

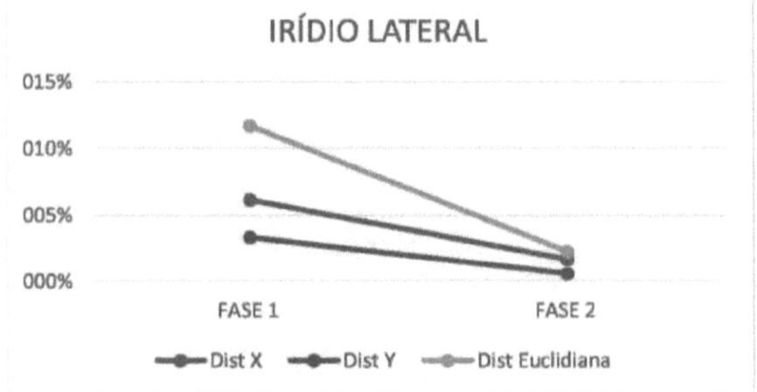

Graph 16: Percentage of markings above the 1% IOD error for the Lateral Iridium point for the three parameters analysed (Scale 0-15%).

Table 11: Table referring to the previous graph showing the percentage of markings above the 1% IOD error for the Lateral Iridium point for the three parameters analysed. The far right column shows the relationship between the error obtained in Phase 1 and Phase 2, in percentage, quantifying the reduction (-) or increase (+) in the error when comparing the two.

Lateral Iridium	**Phase 1**	**Phase 2**	**Ratio (%)**
Dx	6,11%	1,64%	-73,16%
Dy	3,33%	0,56%	-83,18%
From	11,67%	2,22%	-80,98%

4.4.9. Medial iridium

Although the error observed in Phase 1 for this analysed point was small (only 8.89% of the markings were made above the 1% IOD error), it can be seen that there was a 68.73% reduction after using the photoanthropometric description, resulting in an error rate of 2.78% in Phase 2.

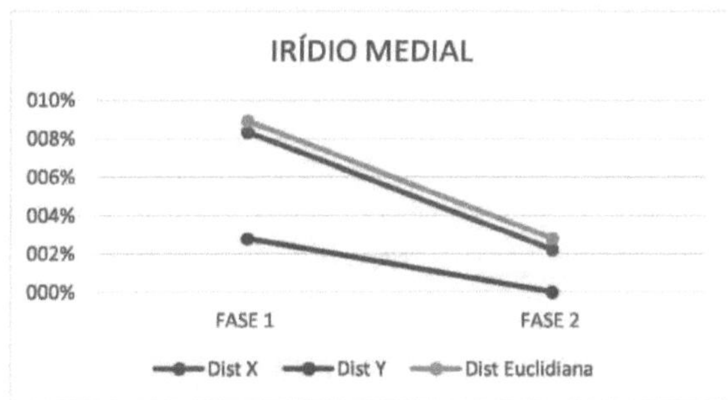

Graph 17: Percentage of markings above the 1% IOD error for the Medial Iridium point for the three parameters analysed (Scale 0-10%).

Table 12: Table referring to the previous graph showing the percentage of markings above the 1% IOD error for the Medial Iridium point for the three parameters analysed. The far right column shows the relationship between the error obtained in Phase 1 and Phase 2, in percentage, quantifying the reduction (-) or increase (+) in the error when comparing the two.

Medial Iridium	**Phase 1**	**Phase 2**	**Ratio (%)**
Dx	8,33%	2,22%	-73,35%
Dy	2,78%	0,00%	-100,00%
From	8,89%	2,78%	-68,73%

4.4.10. Lower Labial

Analysing the graph and table below, it can be seen that there was a 13.05% reduction in the error of the markings in Phase 2 compared to Phase 1, with a small increase in the error for the Dy parameter. Despite the small reduction in error in Phase 2 for this point, 55.56% of the markings were still below the 1% error in this phase.

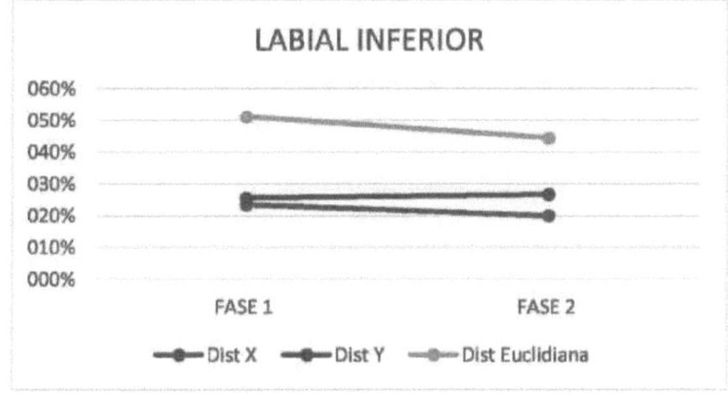

Graph 18: Percentage of markings above the 1% IOD error for the lower lip point for the three parameters analysed (Scale 0-60%).

Table 13: Table referring to the previous graph showing the percentage of markings above the 1% IOD error for the lower lip point for the three parameters analysed. The far right column shows the relationship between the error obtained in Phase 1 and Phase 2, in percentage, quantifying the reduction (-) or increase (+) in the error when comparing the two.

Lower lip	Phase 1	Phase 2	Ratio (%)
Dx	23,33%	20,00%	-14,27%
Dy	25,56%	26,67%	+4,16%
From	51,11%	44,44%	-13,05%

4.4.11. Upper Labial

Analysing the graph and table below, it can be seen that there was a 44.82% reduction in the error in marking the upper lip point after using the photoanthropometric description. Analysing Phase 2, 64.44% of the markings were below the 1% error of the interpupillary distance of the images, compared to 35.56% of the markings made in Phase 1.

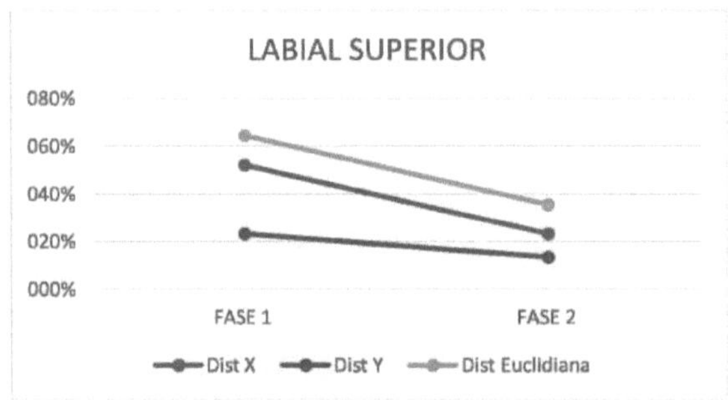

Graph 19: Percentage of markings above the 1% IOD error for the upper lip point for the three parameters analysed (Scale 0-80%).

Table 14: Table referring to the previous graph showing the percentage of markings above the 1% IOD error for the upper lip point for the three parameters analysed. The far right column shows the relationship between the error obtained in Phase 1 and Phase 2, in percentage, quantifying the reduction (-) or increase (+) in the error when comparing the two.

Upper lip	Phase 1	Phase 2	Ratio (%)
Dx	52,22%	23,33%	-55,32%
Dy	23,33%	13,33%	-42,86%

From	64,44%	35,56%	-44,82%

4.4.12. Labiomental

For the Labiomental point, it can be seen that only 21.11% of the markings made in Phase 1 were below the error of 1% of the interpupillary distance of the images, while for Phase 2 there was a small increase in the error (1.39%), resulting in 20% of the markings being made below the error in this phase. There was an increase in error of 4.68% in Dx when comparing both phases.

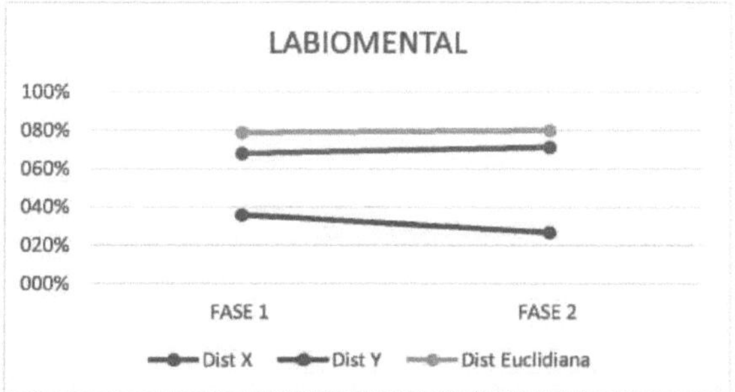

Graph 20: Percentage of markings above the 1% IOD error for the Labiomental point for the three parameters analysed (Scale 0-100%).

Table 15: Table referring to the previous graph showing the percentage of markings above the 1% IOD error for the Labiomental point for the three parameters analysed. The far right column shows the relationship between the error obtained in Phase 1 and Phase 2, in percentage, quantifying the reduction (-) or increase (+) in the error when comparing the two.

Labiomental	**Phase 1**	**Phase 2**	**Ratio (%)**
Dx	67,78%	71,11%	+4,68%
Dy	35,56%	26,67%	-25,00%
From	78,89%	80,00%	+1,39%

4.4.13. Násio

Analysing the graph and table for the nasion point, it can be seen that there was a 90.12% reduction in marking error after using the photoanthropometric description. Analysing Phase 2, 91.11% of the markings were below the error of 1% of the interpupillary distance of the images, compared to 10% of the markings made in Phase 1.

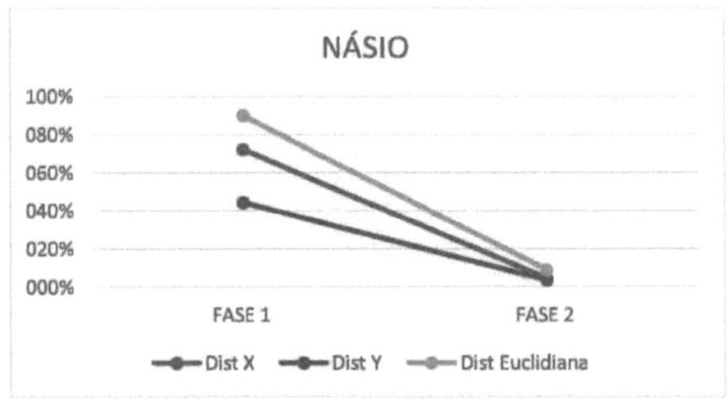

Graph 21: Percentage of markings above the 1% IOD error for the Nasio point for the three parameters analysed (Scale 0-100%).

Table 16: Table referring to the previous graph showing the percentage of markings above the 1% IOD error for the Nasio point for the three parameters analysed. The far right column shows the relationship between the error obtained in Phase 1 and Phase 2, in percentage, quantifying the reduction (-) or increase (+) in the error when comparing the two.

Násio	**Phase 1**	**Phase 2**	**Ratio (%)**
Dx	72,22%	4,44%	-93,85%
Dy	44,44%	3,33%	-92,51%
From	90,00%	8,89%	-90,12%

4.4.14. Stomium

For the Stomium point, 68.89% of the markings made in Phase 1 were below the 1% error of the interpupillary distance of the images, while for Phase 2 there was a decrease in the error (7.14%), resulting in 71.11% of the markings being made below the error in this phase. Despite the increase in Dy error (12.02%), when comparing both phases, all the markings were made below 1% error for Dx, after the photoanthropometric description.

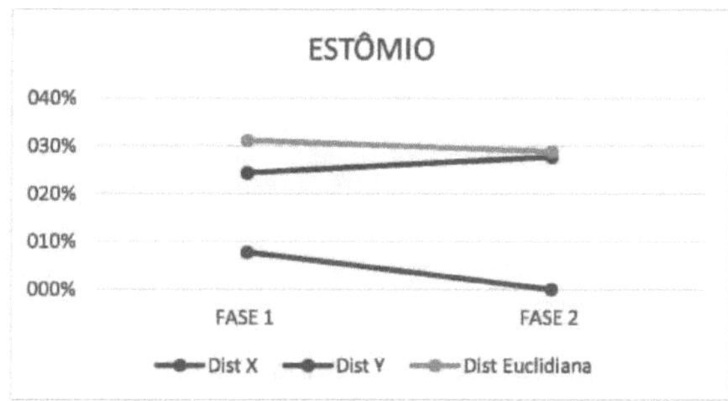

Graph 22: Percentage of markings above the 1% IOD error for the Stomium point for the three parameters analysed (Scale 0-40%).

Table 17: Table referring to the previous graph showing the percentage of markings above the 1% IOD error for the Stomium point for the three parameters analysed. The far right column shows the relationship between the error obtained in Phase 1 and Phase 2, in percentage, quantifying the reduction (-) or increase (+) in the error when comparing the two.

Stomach	**Phase 1**	**Phase 2**	**Ratio (%)**
Dx	7,78%	0,00%	-100,00%
Dy	24,44%	27,78%	+12,02%
From	31,11%	28,89%	-7,14%

4.4.15. Subnasal

For the Subnasal point, it can be seen that 75.56% of the markings made in Phase 1 were below the 1% error of the interpupillary distance of the images, compared to 77.78% of the markings in Phase 2, showing a 9.08% reduction in marking error when comparing both phases. Despite the reduction in error in Dx (55.6%), this point showed an increase in error for Dy (21.47%).

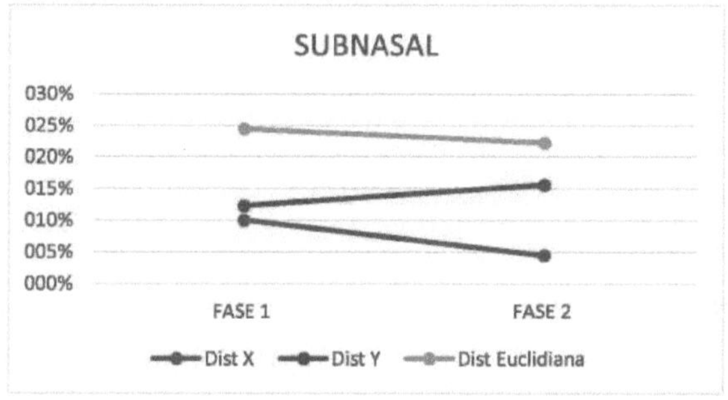

Graph 23: Percentage of markings above the 1% IOD error for the Subnasal point for the three parameters analysed (Scale

0-30%).

Table 18: Table referring to the previous graph showing the percentage of markings above the 1% IOD error for the Subnasal point for the three parameters analysed. The far right column shows the relationship between the error obtained in Phase 1 and Phase 2, in percentage, quantifying the reduction (-) or increase (+) in the error when comparing the two.

Subnasal	Phase 1	Phase 2	Ratio (%)
Dx	10,00%	4,44%	-55,60%
Dy	12,22%	15,56%	+21,47%
From	24,44%	22,22%	-9,08%

4.4.16. Zygian

Analysing the graph and table for the Zygian point, it can be seen that there was a 17.64% reduction in marking error after using the photoanthropometric description. Analysing Phase 1, 5.56% of the markings were below the error of 1% of the interpupillary distance of the images, compared to 22.22% of the markings made in Phase 2. The percentage reduction in error was greater for Dy (91.31%), compared to 17.68% for Dx.

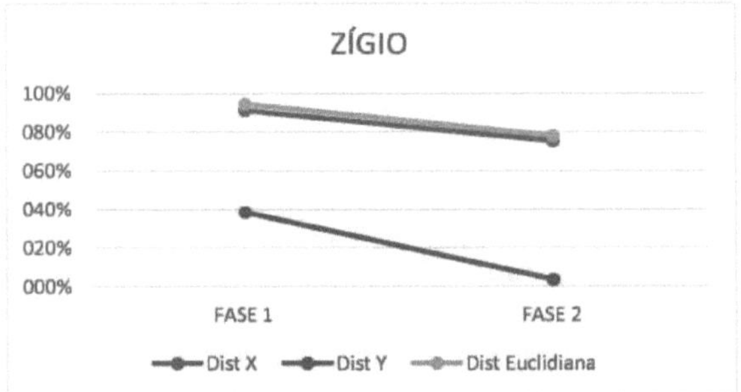

Graph 24: Percentage of markings above the 1% IOD error for the Zygian point for the three parameters analysed (Scale 0-100%).

Table 19: Table referring to the previous graph showing the percentage of markings above the 1% IOD error for the Zygian point for the three parameters analysed. The far right column shows the relationship between the error obtained in Phase 1 and Phase 2, in percentage, quantifying the reduction (-) or increase (+) in the error when comparing the two.

Zygia n	Phase 1	Phase 2	Ratio (%)
Dx	91,11%	75,00%	-17,68%
Dy	38,33%	3,33%	-91,31%

Fro m	94,44%	77,78%	-17,64%

4.5. *Intra-examiner analysis*

The Wilcoxon test showed that there was no difference in the vast majority of markings made by the same examiners in both phases, demonstrating that there was no significant sample evidence to reject the null hypothesis. However, some points showed statistical evidence to affirm that the examiners marked differently for some of the parameters analysed. In Phase 1, two examiners made statistically different markings for the Lateral Iridium point in the Dy parameter and one examiner for the same point but for the De parameter. Also in the same phase, one examiner made different markings for each of the following points and their respective parameters: Zygium (Dy), Medial Iridium (Dy), Gonion (Dy) and Ectocanthion (Dy). In Phase 2, there were more statistically different markings: for the Endocanthion point, two examiners, one for the Dy parameter and one for the De parameter; for the Gonion point, two examiners, one for the Dx parameter and one for the De parameter; and one examiner for each of the points Ectocanthion (Dy), Glabella (Dy), Gnathion (Dy), Lower Labial (Dy), Subnasal (Dx), Upper Labial (Dy), Medial Iridium (Dx), Labiomental (Dx), Lateral Iridium (De) and Zygium (Dy).

CHAPTER 6

Discussion

Facial analyses on photographs have attracted the interest of the scientific community worldwide as an alternative method to direct facial analysis. As it is a two-dimensional representation of a three-dimensional structure that makes up the human face, information about its structures is often lost due to the lack of representation of facial depth and dynamics (STAVRIANOS et al., 2012). This flat, static representation of facial structures ends up restricting their analysis to only the structures that can be seen in the image. As most facial analysis methods were developed taking into account direct access to the subjects being examined, these methodologies generate major difficulties when it comes to applying them to images (STAVRIANOS et al., 2012).

A major demand from forensic and public security organisations worldwide is the comparison of facial images for human identification purposes, as they are often the only materials available for analysis (MORETON; MORLEY, 2011). Even when CCTV images are available, the analysis will inevitably be based on two-dimensional images obtained from them. In this sense, establishing methodologies based exclusively on images, as well as analysing the errors inherent in these methods, is extremely important if they are to be applicable in forensic practice. However, there are few scientific publications that corroborate the needs of these organisations.

In principle, one of the great challenges of facial analyses on images consists of adapting existing cephalometric methodologies so that they can be applied to images. As with any other process, and in order for their relationships to be studied and mapped in a systematic and universal way, it is necessary to standardise the analysis tools, namely the cephalometric points. These have not yet been redefined for use in photoanthropometry, a process that occurred naturally with craniometric points for their application in cephalometry (cephalometric points). The redefinition of these points is necessary because their initial definition makes it difficult or even impossible to determine them in images (YOSHINO et al., 2002).

Photoanthropometry is the science of obtaining measurements through the use of precise anatomical points in various regions of the face or non-specific anatomical areas, as they are visualised in photographs (STAVRIANOS et al., 2012). Although the very definition of the method considers the use of "precise anatomical points", it was possible to observe by analysing the results of this study that the use of the current definition in the literature does not allow these points to be marked precisely. Photoanthropometric analyses are influenced by a myriad of factors, such as those related to the dynamic morphology of the face, its individuality, the angular difference of the camera and the individual's pose, facial expressions, noise in the image and the subjectivity of measuring anatomical reference points (DIBEKLIOGLU, 2012). Therefore, regardless of the method used and however precise it may be, the pattern of facial markings is unlikely to be the same for different facial images, even when considering images of the same individual.

A fundamental point for facial identification methods to be established through photoanthropometric analysis is to survey the influence of each of these factors in this process, so that human variability can be distinguished from the technical variability resulting from image acquisition and the variability arising from the analyses themselves. This knowledge will make it possible to determine acceptable errors for facial image analyses, contributing to the value of this expert evidence and its correct application. Although photoanthropometric studies are based on scientific and objective grounds, the process of comparison and the conclusion of an identification considered to be absolute are explicitly subjective. Initially, the examiner must recognise the anatomical reference points on the face and, from these, facial relationships can be surveyed and compared metrically (DAVIS; VALENTINE; DAVIS, 2010; Í§CAN; LOTH, 2000; KAU et al., 2007; STAVRIANOS et al., 2012). These

Relationships must be compared by observing the sporadicity of their presence in the population under study, at which point an estimate of their random occurrence is made. The more coincidences are found between two patterns being analysed, the greater the conviction among scientists and laypeople that this compatibility cannot be attributed to chance (STONEY, 1991).

The specificity of the characteristics is presented taking into account the circumstances and the population characteristics being analysed. The collection of population data on the presence of certain characteristics is the basis for making reasonable inferences and critical judgements (STONEY, 1991). For objective individuality to be determined, rather than specificity, probabilities would have to be tested and reproduced in a population of hundreds of millions of people. In practical reality, what happens is the application of scientific, critical, expert and enlightened judgement to the determination of a subjective identity (STONEY, 1991).

The terms Photoanthropometry and Photogrammetry have been defined as synonyms in many studies

(HALBERSTEIN, 2001; MORETON; MORLEY, 2011; RAMANATHAN; CHELLAPPA, 2006; WILKINSON; EVANS, 2009). The word "Photogrammetry" has Greek origins and means light, description and measurements (HOUAISS, 2009). It is defined as the art, science and technology of extracting reliable information about physical objects and the environment, such as their shape, position and dimension for the creation of a three-dimensional object-space through processes of recording, measuring and interpreting images; patterns of radiant electromagnetic energy; among other phenomena (ASPRS, 2013; PATIAS, 2002). They are generally used by scientific areas investigating two-dimensional images of geological and architectural structures for their three-dimensional reconstruction (PATIAS, 2002). Some authors also differentiate Photogrammetry - defining it as the process of obtaining measurements by means of images - from Stereophotogrammetry, the latter being conceptualised as the process of obtaining measurements from two-dimensional images in order to obtain information for the three-dimensional reconstruction of a scene (DOUGLAS, 2004).

When used by anthropologists, the term Photogrammetry often refers to measurements on images (ALLANSON, 1997; FARKAS, 1994; GUYOT et al., 2003). Although some methods do not aim for three-dimensional reconstruction using two-dimensional images and do not use objects and the environment as a source of analysis, its definition has been transferred to the medical and anthropological fields and the use of this term has persisted over the years (MITCHELL; NEWTON, 2002). Bearing in mind that the conceptual differentiation between the two lies in the purpose for which they are carried out and their object of analysis, taking these factors into account is fundamental to defining the method in question. When analysing the proportions of facial images, without the aim of obtaining a three-dimensional object-space, the term Photoanthropometry is more appropriate.

Problems related to variability in the marking of anatomical reference points, such as difficulty in visualising and locating some facial structures, overlapping anatomical references and individual variations in the determination of these points can be minimised by redefining them (GIL et al., 2004). The nasion point, for example, has the following craniometric anatomical definition: "Point where the internasal suture and the frontonasal suture meet. It corresponds to the root of the nose." (PEREIRA; ALVIM, 1979). This definition makes it difficult, if not impossible, to accurately determine this point in facial topography. Although the description appears to be sufficient for determining this point on the skull, this statement is not true when analysing the soft tissues of the face, nor on facial images. The lack of definition parameters for photoanthropometry ends up making the marking subjective, contributing to greater variability in the measurement of these points. As a result, areas of application that depend on greater precision in analyses (such as forensics) end up using even more subjective methodologies. An example of this is the consolidated recommendation in favour of morphological analysis when comparing facial images for the purposes of facial identification (FISWG, 2012).

Considering the "classic" *cephalometric definition of* the nasion point (GEORGE, 2007; KOLAR; SALTER, 1997; CATTANEO et al., 2012; ZIMBLER; HAM, 2005), defined as *the "apex of the frontonasal angle",* facial analyses of frontal images create difficulties in measuring it. Not because it is difficult to visualise (as would be the case for some of the cephalometric points used in this study, such as the Zygian and Ectocanthion points, which can be covered by hair or eyelashes, respectively), but because the determination is influenced by the examiner's direct analysis and the standard used in their assessment (profile or frontal). Although these difficulties have been observed by authors who have attempted to analyse facial methodologies in frontal images, they have been unable to clearly define the craniometric points used, which casts doubt on the reproducibility and objectivity of these studies (ASKU; KAYA; KOCADERELI, 2010; DOUGLAS; MUTSVANGWA, 2010; MORETON; MORLEY, 2011).

Determining the *accuracy of* reference points is unfeasible in photoanthropometric analyses because there is no location that can be attributed as correct or true. To this end, a detailed description was sought so that they could be determined as accurately as possible, i.e. with reproducibility. The precision of a method expresses the degree to which the measured quantity is consistent with its mean, making it possible to visualise the dispersion of the markings (MIKHAIL; ACKERMANN, 1976) and the proximity between them, obtained by repeating the measurement process (ZAR, 1999). To determine precision, statistical measures of imprecision (standard deviation) and a measure of data dispersion or random error are recommended, as used to analyse the data in this study (ZAR, 1999).

In facial comparison analyses for human identification purposes, photoanthropometry can be used to metrically compare the relationships of measurements, proportions, angles and indices of one photograph with another, in an attempt to find quantitative visual differences and similarities (DAVIS; VALENTINE; DAVIS, 2010; İÇCAN; LOTH, 2000; KAU et al., 2007; STAVRIANOS et al., 2012). Although not recommended by international organisations due to the lack of studies in the area (FISWG, 2011; 2012; SWGIT, 2004), photoanthropometry has been used as an image comparison technique for over 15 years in UK courts, mainly for exclusion purposes. Furthermore, the number of reports issued in this area has been growing annually (MORETON; MORLEY, 2011). Despite its limitations, the persistent use of photoanthropometric methods by police organisations worldwide indicates the need for more objective practices in this analysis. Wilkinson and Evans (2009) report that the majority of facial image comparison specialists in the UK use a combination of morphological and proportion comparisons, rather than photoanthropometry alone.

The vast majority of existing non-forensic studies seek to establish a correlation between real measurements, obtained directly from the individual, and those obtained indirectly through images, in order to check that the proportions are maintained. These studies end up establishing measurement error limits, within which measurement variability can be classified as acceptable, as well as the angles obtained from them. Linear or angular measurements greater than these values would be considered high and significant absolute errors. Some of these studies consider a reliability value of one millimetre to be acceptable for linear measurements (FARKAS, 1994, 1996; ASKU 2010; COLOMBO, 2004; CUMMINS; BISHARA; JAKOBSEN, 1995; BISHARA; JORGENSEN; JAKOBSEN, 1998; STRAUSS et al., 1997). Rakosi (1982) and Farkas; Bryson; Klotz (1980) suggest that an error of two millimetres can be considered acceptable, while Forsyth and Davis (1996) and Richardson (1981) consider an error of one millimetre to be desirable. For angular measurements, reliability is determined within an error of 1° (CUMMINS; BISHARA; JAKOBSEN, 1995), 1.5° (COLOMBO, 2004) or 2° (FARKAS, 1994; STRAUSS et al., 1997), depending on the study. Despite the importance of this data for various areas of knowledge, the survey of variability between direct and indirect measurements is not of great relevance in the forensic field, since in the vast majority of cases the physical presence of the examinee is impractical. However, its precepts can lead to a better understanding of facial analyses on images. The present study, considering a limit of 2.61 pixels (1% of the IOD), established a distance corresponding to 0.65 mm in vivo as the error threshold, a lower limit than that recommended by these studies.

Analysing horizontal distance and vertical distance separately is extremely important when using indices, as greater variations on the "y" axis have a greater influence on the results for certain points, while for others, greater variations on the "x" axis are more significant. The study by Çeliktutan; Ulukaya; Sankur (2013) did not analyse the distances separately, probably because they were vector analyses, which are widely used for automated determination of anatomical reference points. It can be seen that the maximum error of 10%, established as acceptable for automated determination studies (ÇELIKTUTAN; ULUKAYA; SANKUR, 2013; DIBEKLIOGLU, 2012), is greater than what would be acceptable for manual analyses, the vast majority of whose values were below the 1% error after adopting the methodology proposed in this study. The 5% error also proved to be large for these analyses, as 100% of the markings were below this index. Studies that examine errors smaller than 5% would be important in order to visualise the behaviour of markings when classified into smaller intervals (errors of 4%, 3%, 2% and 0.5%).

In an attempt to get round the problems arising from the description of the anatomical points used as a reference in establishing facial relationships, some studies have resorted to direct marking on the face prior to taking the photographs in order to collect data on the variability of measurements between images (FARKAS, 1994; GUYURON, 1988; PURKAIT, 2004), or even prior visual inspection to help determine the reference points on the images (COLOMBO, 2004). The demarcated faces were then photographed and lines, angles and frontal and lateral measurements were established for future variability analyses. Although it makes it possible to scale the photograph for standardised analyses, which are closer to the actual size of the individual, its application is also hampered when direct analysis is impossible.

A common situation in facial images, sources of forensic comparison, is the lack of scales or comparison standards, requiring the use of reference distances so that they can be standardised (STAVRIANOS et al., 2012). Images are generally normalised in order to correct their positioning in terms of rotation, translation and scaling, and only after this can they be compared with each other (MACHADO et al., 2014). Some studies have observed better results when using the Endocanthion-Endocanthion (en-en) normalisation measure (FARKAS; BRYSON; KLOTZ, 1980). In the study by Asku et al. (2010), however, the Ectocanthion-Ectocanthion (ex-ex) and Endocanthion-Endocanthion (en-en) normalisation distances proved to be equally reliable. It should be noted that the Federal Police generally use the interpupillary distance for this function (MACHADO et al., 2014). In this study, as standardised images were used, only translation adjustments were made. To analyse the error, the interpupillary distance was used as described by Çeliktutan; Ulukaya; Sankur (2013). According to Dibeklioglu (2012), this distance is a reliable measure because it provides a constant value in terms of scale, making it the most widely used measure for calculating marking error in two-dimensional images.

Once the images have been standardised, the examiner has various means of analysis available for facial mapping, including: analysis of facial proportions; quantitative analysis of linear measurements, as well as angles and indices obtained from them; analysis of Facial Geometry; and analysis of the pattern of arrangement of anatomical reference points.

In principle, all these tools can be used for this purpose. However, the lack of population surveys and studies on the interference of external factors in the variability of these analyses hinders the forensic application of most of them, leading, in practice, to a predilection for analyses of proportions (MACHADO et al., 2014). According to Steele (2013), the study of facial proportions should be carried out initially and as a form of exclusion. If these relationships are compatible or their incompatibility is justified, the study should be analysed more faithfully using measurements (STEELE, 2013). In analysing proportions, the face is initially divided into thirds using two horizontal planes - the transverse nasal plane, which passes through the Subnasal point and divides the face into two portions - and the transglabellar plane - which passes through the Glabella point and defines the upper limit of the face - and then into fifths using six vertical planes that pass through the Zygian, Ectocanthion and Endocanthion points on both sides of the face (MACHADO et al., 2014; STEELE, 2013).

Other vertical and horizontal reference lines can be included in the analyses to help study the proportions and compatibility between them (STEELE, 2013). Mismatches in the lower vertical third can be explained by the loss of the vertical dimension of occlusion due to tooth wear or loss, especially when the comparison is made using images with a long acquisition interval. Generally, the vertical fifths are only analysed when there is compatibility for comparing the vertical thirds (STEELE, 2013). Although the variability in the determination of anatomical points is not so critical in analyses of proportions, as it does not take into account quantitative comparison values and is more related to morphological analyses than to photoanthropometric analyses as such, the systematisation of these determinations is interesting in terms of standardising analyses and the reliable exchange of information.

Linear measurements are distances obtained by joining any two reference points (KLEINBERG, 2008). In principle, in this study, it would be possible to produce 552 linear measurements (24 x 23) using the 24 photoanthropometric points (KLEINBERG, 2008). However, of all these measurements, a subset must be selected, especially if these measurements are to be used to determine indices or angles, the latter being 304,152 possible combinations in this study (552 x 551) (KLEINBERG, 2008). These measurements can be unilateral or bilateral. Among the linear measurements that can be established are: mandibular width (gogo); facial height (n-gn); upper facial height (n-sto); lateral facial height (ex-go); intercanthal width (en-en); biocular width (ex-ex); ocular fissure length (en-ex); nasal width (al-al); labial width (ch-ch) (KOLAR; SALTER,1997). The most relevant in image comparisons for human identification purposes are the horizontal distances: intercanthal (en-en), interpupillary distance, labial width (ch-ch) and nasal width (al-al) (STEELE, 2013). These measurements show less variation with the individual's age and in relation to other factors, such as weight loss or gain (STEELE, 2013). Kleinberg (2008) considered ex-n and ex-sto distances to be important because the related points are less affected by facial expression. As this is a quantitative analysis, it is extremely important that the measurements are established accurately. Ideally, the markings should be made in the same place on both photographs. In this sense, it is imperative to standardise this analysis and the reference points (STEELE, 2013).

In cases where absolute values cannot be obtained from images due to the lack of scales, a photoanthropometric tool available is the use of indices (STEELE, 2013). Generally, these indices are calculated by the ratio between each distance obtained between any two points and the greatest distance available from the same plane. This gives the facial height (n-gn) as the maximum vertical measurement and the facial width (zn-zn) as the maximum horizontal measurement, multiplied by 100 (STAVRIANOS et al., 2012). All the measurements taken are converted into indices and compared to each other. However, due to the lack of studies in the area, acceptable error values for determining an identification or exclusion, or for data to be designated as inconclusive, are unknown. This factor ends up limiting the use of indices in human identification, with some authors recommending them only for the exclusion of individuals (MORETON; MORLEY, 2011; STAVRIANOS et al., 2012). According to Steele (2013), the best accepted difference in indices for determining compatibility would be around 0.5%. However, this has not been scientifically confirmed.

For human identification to be carried out using a pattern of facial points, it is necessary to collect population data in order to establish the facial pattern of the population under study, the probability of occurrence of a certain analysed characteristic and the probability of including this pattern in the sample. While the facial characteristics of the population of interest have not been surveyed, photoanthropometric points are of great importance so that facial relationships can be surveyed and compared using the analyses already reported, as well as geometric figures, masks or templates using the Facial Geometry Technique (MACHADO et al., 2014).

Regardless of the analysis carried out in comparisons of facial images for human identification purposes, standardisation of the technique, homogenisation of the reference points and the universality of their determination are essential for the advancement of studies in this area and for reliable quantitative analysis methods to be established. This study showed that, although based on the same initial anatomical description, a description used by studies in various areas, the average variability in the markings of the anatomical reference points in the first phase was five times greater than the average variability in the second phase, based on the standard deviation. The definition of cephalometric landmarks in the literature does not allow for the reproducibility of these landmarks on frontal images. There is a need for a better description and standardisation of these landmarks so that, regardless of the science that uses them or the professional, these landmarks can be uniquely identified when defined in a wide variety of areas. This aspect is even more important when they are used in forensic sciences, as reproducing the data is fundamental to characterising the objectivity so sought after in human identification methods.

Prior to using the description proposed in this study, it can be seen that the examiners had difficulty determining the Gonion point, corroborating the studies by Colombo (2004), Farkas; Bryson; Klotz (1980) and Asku; Kaya; Kocadereli (2010). This difficulty was evidenced by the greater variability of this point in the three parameters analysed, compared to the other points, thus indicating the need to establish a more detailed definition, especially with regard to determining a vertical anatomical reference. The Zygian, Glabella and Nasion points, together with the Gonion, were among the four points with the greatest variability in all the parameters analysed. These points are of great importance for surveying linear measurements, as well as in the use of cephalometric indices such as the Facial Index, the Upper Facial Index and the Nasal Index, thus denoting the subjectivity of their measurement (ARBENZ, 1988).

In forensic anthropometry, Facial Index data is used to establish an individual's ancestry. The Facial Index is obtained by dividing the facial height (n- gn) by the facial width (zn-zn), with the quotient multiplied by 100 (FARKAS, 1994; FARKAS; MUNRO, 1987). Individuals with long faces, known as dolichocephalics and predominantly Caucasian, have indices of less than 75.9 (ENLOW; POSTON; BAKOR, 1993). Breeds with medium faces have indices between 76 and 80.9 and breeds with short faces, or brachycephalics, common among North American Indians, Orientals and blacks (PROFITT; AKERMAN, 1996), have indices higher than 81 (ENLOW; HANS, 1996). Considering the correspondence observed in the study of approximately four pixels for each millimetre of the face, as well as the variability observed, we can conclude that a lack of precision in determining the nasion point, for example, would be enough to include an individual in a different racial classification. Considering that the average dispersion in pixels from this point to

Dy (determinant of the vertical variation) was 37.475, equivalent to approximately nine millimetres on the face. This dispersion would be sufficient for a Caucasian individual to be considered oriental. Analysing the variation, in pixels, of the Ionian point presented for De (212.305) - a distance that represents the real distance formed by the union of the two points determined - it would denote 53 millimetres in the person *in vivo,* an unacceptable variability for any study area.

When the analyses are carried out by the same examiners or when they have been calibrated beforehand, systematisation is less complex to achieve. This form of analysis is carried out in some studies in order to reduce the variability of determinations resulting from different examiners (ASKU; KAYA; KOCADERELI, 2010; COLOMBO, 2004; CUMMINS; BISHARA; JAKOBSEN, 1995). This study found that the vast majority of markings made by the same examiners in both phases were statistically the same, according to each point and parameter analysed. However, in the second phase there were more points with different markings, contradicting these studies in the sense that analysis by the same examiner reduces measurement variability. Bearing in mind that accuracy in determining reference points depends on the examiner's disposition, their degree of tiredness and how many analyses were carried out in a single day, this result may have occurred because these markings were carried out on the last day of the analyses, after four days of markings (KLEINBERG, 2008). Despite the breaks and intervals given between markings, this factor may have contributed to a reduction in the examiners' attention span. In cases of facial identification, the determination of anatomical reference points is carried out by different professionals from a wide range of backgrounds, a factor that drives the development of methodologies that - regardless of the examiner - achieve similar results.

The standardisation methodology proposed for marking the anatomical reference points on frontal photographs was presented in the form of a manual (Appendix A) and initially consisted of a presentation of the SMVFace programme interfaces and an operational description of the commands and tools needed for proper handling when marking these points. Some of these tools were designed to be inserted after marking specific points, such as the centre of the pupil and the eye circumference, which appear after determining the four Iridium points (two for each hemiface) and the orbital midline, determined after marking the contralateral Ectocanthion and Endocanthion points. Due to the non-existence or difficulty in visualising the anatomical reference structures in the frontal norm, the establishment of these tools introduced greater objectivity into the analysis by creating marking references, thus reducing the individual interpretation of the examiners as to their proper location.

As the Glabella point is located between the superciliary arches and these, in turn, are just above the cranial orbital cavities, it is difficult to determine in frontal images. The introduction of the ocular circumference tool made it possible to create a reference close to the anatomical position of the orbit and to visualise its upper portion which, together with the use of the horizontal reference line, made it possible to determine this point more carefully and objectively. Using this methodology, the centre of the pupil (an extremely important reference point for standardising and scaling comparison source images) was automatically established after determining the Iridium points, thus eliminating subjectivity in its measurement. The orbital midline was referred to in this way so as not to give rise to a relationship with the facial midline, because although both divide the face into two hemifaces, the former was designed for use in facial images and its determination is influenced by the determination of the Ectocanthion and Endocanthion points, unlike the facial midline (MACHADO et al., 2014).

Horizontal and vertical reference lines were included in the analyses to make it easier to visualise the point itself (by intersecting the two) and the ends of the structures (by visualising the point of tangency). The manual also contains, for each analysis point: a photoanthropometric description using visually identifiable references in frontal images; operating procedures for marking each specific point, with a detailed and successive explanation of each necessary step; and illustrations of their location on the facial topography. A reference labial midline was created, automatically inserted after determining the bilateral Chelion points, distinct from the orbital midline. This distinction was made in order not to exclude from the analysis the anatomical diversity of the lips observed in the study population. Using the orbital midline - instead of the labial midline - to determine the Stomal and Lower Labial points would concentrate these determinations in the central region of the image, cancelling out the individuality of the lip patterns observed. Similarly, it has been observed that the insertion of the points of the Crista Filtral (point of the apex of the cupid's bow) in future analyses may be interesting in recording this individuality (KOLAR; SALTER,1997).

The choice of points used in this analysis was based mainly on their visualisation and variability. In this way, points with greater variability - such as the eyebrow points - and points easily covered by facial structures - such as the Trichion and Eurio, which are usually covered by the individual's hair - were removed from the analysis (PEREIRA; ALVIM, 1979).

As for analysing the pattern of anatomical reference points, as described above, although the use of a small number of points does not provide sufficient data for facial identification, there are four points in particular that may be more beneficial than others. These are: the two Ectocanthions, the Stomach and the Nasion (KLEINBERG, 2008). These points showed extremely favourable results in this study after their redefinition, demonstrating an average variability of 0.96 mm, 0.58 mm and 0.15 mm, respectively. According to the author, the Ectocanthion and Nasion points remain relatively fixed to facial expressions, while for the

Stomal point, its importance is more related to the relative ease of marking it, a situation that was corroborated in the second phase of this study (KLEINBERG, 2008).

The standardisation proposed through the establishment of structural and topographical references that can only be seen in the images, as well as the operational description of the method, led to a significant reduction in the average dispersion for practically all the points (highly significant for the Alar, Endocanthion, Glabella, Gonion, Medial Iridium, Labial Superior and Zygium points; significant, in turn, for the Lateral Iridium, Nasion and Subnasal points), indicating that the proposed methodology is valid for increasing the accuracy of examiners when marking anatomical reference points. However, the same anatomical and operational description adopted in the second phase of this study increased the dispersion in the determination of some points such as Chelion, Gnathion and Labial Inferior. It can be concluded from this data that the description used in the second phase was not adequate enough to improve accuracy, and that further refinement of the description is needed. A summary of each specific point is presented below.

For the Alar point, the result was extremely favourable, showing a highly significant reduction in variability after adopting the photoanthropometric description for all the parameters analysed, resulting in an average variability of 0.3 mm, much lower than the error limit considered acceptable between direct and indirect measurements (FARKAS, 1994, 1996; ASKU 2010; COLOMBO, 2004; CUMMINS; BISHARA; JAKOBSEN, 1995; BISHARA; JORGENSEN; JAKOBSEN, 1998; STRAUSS et al., 1997). This result was achieved despite the difficulties inherent to facial analysis based exclusively on images, unlike the studies that considered measurements obtained directly from the individual as one side of the comparison. Variability was even lower for the most critical parameter, the horizontal reference, with an average value of 0.056 mm. This factor is extremely important given that this point is commonly used to establish horizontal relationships - such as measuring nasal width - and to determine the Nasal Index and the Nose-Face Width Index (ROELOFSE; STEYN; BECKER, 2008).

The Chelion point was one of the points that showed an unfavourable result in this study, as the initial description proved to be more efficient for greater accuracy of the markings than the photoanthropometric description. The average initial dispersion was 0.77 mm, compared to 1.14 mm in the second phase, which was greater for the parameter of greatest interest, the horizontal reference. This result shows that it was more difficult for the examiners to determine "the lateral limit of the labial rima", a definition included in the proposed methodology. This difficulty was probably due to the fact that this region is difficult to visualise because of the frequent presence of shadows. This result corroborates the study by Bishara; Jorgensen; Jakobsen (1998), who observed less reliability in localising this point, also due to the presence of shadows in the buccal angle and lip movement. Despite this increase, most of the markings were made within the lower limit proposed by the study by Çeliktutan; Ulukaya; Sankur (2013) for automated analyses. However, in order to improve the proposed description and reduce the dispersion of the markings, improving the definition is advisable, especially when considering its future use in establishing facial patterns by anatomical localisation of its reference points.

Another point that showed a favourable result was the Ectocanthion, a point that gives rise to a of reference distances for image standardisation and is widely used to determine horizontal measurements and facial indices. Initially, it showed less variability compared to the other points, reducing even further after the photoanthropometric description, reaching an average value of 0.96 mm. There was also a reduction in the error of the markings, as more than half of them were below the minimum error recommended by the study by Çeliktutan; Ulukaya; Sankur (2013).

The Endocanthion point also showed a favourable result, as it had a 65% reduction in measurement variability after the photoanthropometric description was adopted, determining an average value of 0.42 mm. Consequently, most of the markings were below the 1% IOD error, which corresponds to approximately 0.65 mm of the facial topography. As it is a point used to determine the en-en reference distance, its accuracy is essential if the geometric transformations (translation, rotation and scaling) are to be carried out uniformly on both images being compared. As it is a horizontal reference, the variation in Dx is more critical for this point. However, it showed an even smaller variation for this parameter, around 0.38 mm.

The Stomium point, on the other hand, showed an extremely favourable result. Although the variances were statistically the same for the horizontal parameter (0.74 mm in the first phase and 0.66 mm for the second), there was a reduction of almost 84% in the variability of the markings of this point for the other parameters analysed, resulting in an average variability of 0.58 mm for the Euclidean distance and 0.06 mm for the vertical distance. Although the error was already low in the initial phase, there was a slight reduction in this in Phase 2, placing more than 70% of the markings within a limit of 2.61 pixels (1% of the IOD), which would correspond to a distance of 0.65 mm in vivo. The error for horizontal distances was reduced by 100%, demonstrating that the insertion of the buccal midline was fundamental in establishing a horizontal reference in this determination. These results prove that this point has adequate variability for use in facial comparisons for human identification purposes, from its use for general measurements to the establishment of indices and facial proportions. Further studies are needed to determine the facial pattern, as well as other points that showed low dispersion in their determinations.

The Glabella point showed an extremely favourable result, a circumstance of great relevance since it is used as a reference for surveying vertical facial dimensions (such as facial height, for example) and is included in various facial indices. Inaccurate determination of this point would lead to erroneous qualifications of the group being analysed. This point had the third highest initial variability, especially for the vertical reference, making it a critical point for use in facial analyses using the current description in the world literature, as it would compromise the fidelity of the facial indices that relate to it. After adopting the description proposed in this study, there was a 96% reduction in variability (from 13.19 mm to 0.49 mm), especially with regard to the vertical reference. In addition, the vast majority of markings were below the minimum error of 1% of the ODI.

A relatively unfavourable result was observed for the Gnathio point, which showed an increase of almost 115% in its variability in the second phase, reaching an average value of 2.12 mm. Analysing the parameters separately, there was an increase for the horizontal parameter (from 1.10 mm to 2.26 mm), but there was a significant reduction for the vertical parameter (a parameter of greater interest for use in surveying facial height and determining proportions and indices) (from 0.16 mm to 0.06 mm). These results show that the description is sufficiently adequate for the applications reported, but for surveying facial patterns, the description should be re-evaluated to allow better definition of the horizontal reference structures. In this respect, further studies are also needed to define suitable variabilities and the number of compatibilities needed to determine an identification.

One factor that may have contributed to this dispersion was leaving the decision of whether or not to use the orbital midline to the examiner, as described below: "When the chin has no lower point, because it has a more rectilinear shape, the orbital midline should be used as a reference for marking this point. When there is a greater projection (noticeable enough to say that it is a personal characteristic) and it is possible to define a lower point, the orbital midline should not be considered." For those who opted to use the orbital midline, the variability in determining the Lateral Iridium and Medial Iridium points (points that define the positioning of this line) may have contributed to greater variability in the horizontal parameter of this point. Contrary to expectations, the presence of the "jowl" was not the main element in the measurement variability, because if it were, the variability in the vertical parameter would have been greater. Considering also that, after the description, more than half of the markings were below the minimum error established for automated analyses, the result for this point was not entirely unfavourable.

With regard to point Gônio, the result was extremely favourable. This point showed the greatest initial variability compared to the other points, especially for vertical distances. After the photoanthropometric description, there was an almost 100 per cent reduction in variability for all parameters. There was also a significant reduction in marking error in the second phase. This reduction can be explained by the fact that the initial description is extremely unfavourable for determining this point in frontal images, as it defines it as "the *point of the angle of the mandible"*, a concept that favours its visualisation in profile analyses. The creation of frontal references to determine this point was fundamental to reducing variability. The Gônio point showed a reduction in average variability from 5.3 cm to 0.25 mm. An even greater reduction was observed when analysing the horizontal parameter separately (0.2 mm), making this point an important reference for determining horizontal distances and for surveying ratio indices.

Another point with an extremely favourable result was Lateral Iridium. This point showed the least variability of all the other points in both phases analysed (0.2 mm for the first phase and 0.09 mm for the second). This result raises particular interest for its inclusion in analyses of proportions, indices and even in the establishment of facial patterns, an interest which, until now, had been of little relevance. Similarly, the average variability presented for the horizontal parameter (0.03 mm) points to its predilection (along with the Medial Iridium point) in standardisation distances when using the proposed methodology. The same considerations can be applied to the

Medial Iridium, as it showed a 90% reduction in the variability of its measurement (from 1.08 mm in the first phase to 0.1 mm in the second), reaching the same value for the horizontal parameter observed for the Lateral Iridium point (0.03 mm). Considering the vertical reference, all the markings were below the IOD's 1% margin of error in this analysis. This factor is probably due to the Lateral Iridium being used as the horizontal reference.

The Lower Labial point showed an unfavourable result. The results showed an 18% increase in the variability of its measurement (resulting in a value of 0.85 mm in the first phase and one millimetre in the second phase). Despite the slight increase in variability, there was a reduction in the error of the markings, placing the vast majority of markings below 1% error. This is a commonly used point for determining vertical linear reference measurements. In this sense, as there was a reduction in variability when analysing this parameter specifically (0.79 mm), the Lower Labial point appears to be reliable for use in establishing ratio relationships, indices and vertical linear measurements.

The upper lip point showed an extremely favourable result. This shows that the description proposed in this study was responsible for reducing the variability in determining this point by almost 82% (from 3.06 mm to one millimetre). The reduction was even greater for the vertical distance, the most critical parameter for this point, generating a value of 0.48 mm. These results make this point suitable for use in establishing proportions, indices and linear distances, especially vertical distances. However, further studies are required for its use in surveying facial patterns.

An unfavourable result was observed for the Labiomental point. Despite the reduction in initial variability (from 5.31 mm to 3.53 mm), this was insufficient to include the markings within the 1% error limit adopted in this study. This shows that the description presented in the proposed methodology was effective in reducing variability, although it should be improved. The use of light transition analysis in the description, as presented - "region of transition between shadow (mentolabial sulcus) and light (projection of the chin)" - may not have brought the desired objectivity to the analysis, as it refers to the presence of this characteristic as the possibility of demarcation.

It should be noted that the mentolabial sulcus, the depression between the lower lip and the mental region on which the Labiomental point is determined, is often not well demarcated, a fact that possibly made it difficult to determine this point, thus allowing subjective interpretations by the examiners. Randomisation in determining the samples did not allow this factor to be controlled. In this way, the variability results were influenced by the characteristics of the study population, most of whom had no demarcated mentolabial sulcus. Given the existence of other facial points that can be used as a vertical reference for analysing linear measurements and indices - and which showed less variability than the Labiomental point - the Subnasal, Stomal and Labial Superior points should be preferred for these analyses.

The nasion point, on the other hand, showed an extremely favourable result for use in facial comparison analyses. This point had the fourth highest initial variability, even higher for the vertical distance, demonstrating that its determination in images based on the current description is critical, especially given that the anatomical references used in the description can be visualised in lateral norm. After the photoanthropometric description, there was a 98% reduction in variability (from 8.08 mm to 0.14 mm), especially in the vertical distance (from 9.36 mm to 0.11 mm), a situation that is extremely favourable for this point, as it makes up, along with the Glabella, the points related to the determination of facial height and the survey of indices and proportions. Consequently, it also showed a significant reduction in error, with almost all of its points remaining within the 1% margin of the IOD.

A favourable result can also be seen for the Subnasal point. The initial variability was three times greater than after the photoanthropometric description (from 1.3 mm to 0.37 mm). Although the error was initially low, with most of the markings made within the 1% limit, a reduction can be seen. This point is widely used to establish nasal height together with the nasion, which is used in indices to determine ancestry. It is also used to establish the limit of the lower facial third in proportion ratios. The results presented show that this point is suitable for application in linear measurements in general, in proportions and in facial indices.

A relatively favourable result was shown by the Zygian point. Initially, this point had the second highest initial variability, with a value of approximately 16.88 mm (considering the Euclidean distance). Despite the reduction of almost 42% in variability and the reduction in the error of the markings after using the photoanthropometric description, this point needs an improvement in the description, as only a small amount of the markings (22.22%) were below the margin of error of 1% of the IOD, indicating that its use for establishing facial patterns is not recommended. Despite the initial high variability in the vertical distance (17.68 mm), this would not extensively jeopardise its use in facial indices, as this point is closely related to horizontal facial distances, especially in establishing facial width, and for this parameter the reduction was significant (from 1.22 mm in the first phase to 0.14 mm). In practice, this point can be used to reliably analyse horizontal relationships, as well as indices that include it as a determinant of facial width. It would be interesting to improve the description by including more markings within the 1% error threshold.

Analysing all the data together, it can be seen that there was a reduction in marking error. From an initial rate of 59.22% of markings above the 1% margin, a rate of 78.82% was observed in the second phase, meaning that almost 80% of markings in the second phase were below an error of 2.61 pixels or 0.65 mm in vivo. Considering the values established as acceptable for studies comparing the variability of direct and image analyses, set at one millimetre (FARKAS, 1994, 1996; ASKU 2010; COLOMBO, 2004; CUMMINS; BISHARA; JAKOBSEN, 1995; BISHARA; JORGENSEN; JAKOBSEN, 1998; STRAUSS et al, 1997) and two millimetres (RAKOSI, 1982; FARKAS; BRYSON; KLOTZ, 1980), depending on the authors, the error obtained in most of the markings was below acceptable error.

A much-discussed factor in photoanthropometric analysis is the multiplicity of knowledge required for its study and the vagueness of the area of knowledge to which it should be assigned. As it encompasses a range of concepts and specifications from various fields of study, its analysis is complex and methodologies must follow the precepts of each area of knowledge. Likewise, it is difficult to establish which professional is best qualified to carry it out, given that it involves knowledge of Anatomy, Anthropology, Photography, Computer Science and Information Technology. Ideally, one should have a basic knowledge of craniofacial anatomy, as well as specific training in locating the photoanthropometric points needed to carry out these analyses. In this study, five examiners with mastery of and experience in craniofacial anatomy took part in the study, in order to exclude variability due to the lack of these skills. Studies that collect data on markings made by examiners with no knowledge of the area would be important to determine the method's reproducibility, regardless of the examiner's experience and training.

The proposal to improve and standardise the frontal facial examination technique on photographic images is of great relevance to facial identification studies, but further studies are needed. Establishing visual references for the location of these cephalometric points is a basic step in making analysis techniques feasible, as it will allow for the standardisation of reference points and lead to the standardisation of the examinations carried out. Achieving this could lead in the future to the development of a "facial impression" method, whereby each individual would have a different arrangement of photoanthropometric points that can be compared and consequently used for human identification. This method would be of great relevance, especially in anti-terrorism policies at airports or even in cases of child pornography, where often only images from video cameras or digital photographs are available for analysis.

Determining anatomical reference points on images can be done automatically and is one of the areas of study in facial biometrics, a term that currently refers mainly to computerised technologies that analyse facial biological data in a database for the purpose of authenticating identities (STEELE, 2013). However, its realisation depends on specific software and the development of algorithms that allow the facial anatomy of images to be read by mapping texture, colour, brightness and so on, culminating in the recording of a digital representation of them. Contrary to what one might imagine, these methods are no better than non-automated identification of an individual (STEELE, 2013).

The problems faced by these systems are the same as those faced by facial analysis on images, such as variation in the angle of the face/camera, lighting, facial expression, the obstruction of visualisation of facial structures (hair, glasses, hat) and the need to have an image for comparison (STEELE, 2013). These systems work with a multitude of anatomical points and, until now, none of the facial biometric methods have been sufficiently accurate at positively identifying the individual without significant human intervention (STEELE, 2013). They are generally used to reduce the number of possible positive identifications so that they can then be analysed by the expert (KLEINBERG, 2008).

As previously reported, the error rate of these methods is high. In facial recognition carried out at airports and borders, by comparing them with standard passport photographs, the error rate is around 15% (KLEINBERG, 2008; STEELE, 2013). In addition, this type of facial recognition requires a previous database with biometrically mapped faces, and many photographs, due to damage or poor image quality, do not allow this process (STEELE, 2013). In fact, they can hardly distinguish similar faces of people from the same family or even recognise faces that are not related in any way. What's more, these methods are expensive and difficult to use, as well as being more likely to result in false identification or false exclusion (KLEINBERG, 2008). The trained human eye, after all, is much more capable of discerning subtle differences and making accurate comparisons (STEELE, 2013).

The use of photoanthropometry in facial comparison processes for human identification purposes is extensively questioned worldwide by police and judicial bodies. This is mainly due to the fact that its applicability is seen only for use in facial indices. Comparing the numerical values of these indices does not express the reliability that these examinations require, not least because, due to the lack of population data, the margin of error of these values is unknown. However, once the error in determining photoanthropometric points is known, facial measurements and ratios can be used for the purposes of population inclusion, exclusion and human identification, depending on the discriminating power of these characteristics, as well as the population being analysed (whether closed or open).

In general, this study shows that there was standardisation and a significant reduction in the average dispersion between observers when determining cephalometric points, allowing for greater reproducibility in the markings and, consequently, greater fidelity in the analyses. Some points, such as Chelion, Gnathion and Labial Inferior, showed unfavourable results for this study, with larger variances in the first phase instead of the second, when the opposite would have been expected. Despite the unsatisfactory results for these points, more than half of the markings were within the error limit of 1% of the IOD in all phases, and are therefore acceptable for the use of photoanthropometric techniques.

However, more studies are needed to improve the description and standardisation of the technique so that accuracy can be achieved regardless of the examiner, the photo being assessed and the cephalometric points. The proposition of an analysis methodology, the standardisation of the base references for obtaining facial relationships, as well as the validation of image analysis methodologies are imperative for scientific development in this area which has great appeal to police and forensic bodies around the world. Automated facial identification systems already recognise facial patterns and compare them to a database. However, the great demand for forensic and police facial analyses consists of examining two-dimensional images, precisely because it is common to have previous records for comparison.

CHAPTER 7

Conclusion

Based on the methodology proposed and the results of this study, it can be concluded that:

F It was possible to improve facial analysis on frontal images by proposing a methodology for standardising cephalometric points, presented in the form of a manual (Manual for marking photoanthropometric points on frontal facial images using SMVFace software - Appendix A);

A The descriptions in the manual proved to be better adapted to markings on photographic images when compared to the "classic" descriptions, as they led to more precise markings on practically all the cephalometric points analysed;

The photoanthropometric points that showed the greatest variability in measurement prior to adopting the proposed methodology, in descending order, were: Gonium, Zygium, Glabella, Nasion, Labiomental, Stomium, Labial Superior, Subnasal, Ectocanthion, Endocanthion, Medial Iridium, Gnathion, Labial Inferior, Alar, Chelion and Lateral Iridium;

The photoanthropometric points that showed the greatest variability in measurement after adopting the proposed methodology, in descending order, were: Zygium, Labiomental, Gnathion, Chelion, Labial Inferior, Ectocanthion, Stomium, Labial Superior, Glabella, Endocanthion, Subnasal, Alar, Gonium, Nasion, Medial Iridium and Lateral Iridium;

The photoanthropometric points that showed the greatest reduction in variability with the adoption of the new methodology, in descending order, were: Gonium, Glabella, Nasion, Zygium, Stomium, Labial Superior, Labiomental, Gnathion, Medial Iridium, Subnasal, Endocanthion, Alar, Chelion, Ectocanthion, Labial Inferior and Lateral Iridium. Some

points showed a reduction in variability of more than 90 per cent, such as Glabela, Gônio, Irídio Medial and Násio;

F Increases in variability were observed for the Chelion, Labial Inferior and Gnathion points. Despite this, most of the markings for these points were made below the 1% IOD error, considered acceptable by some studies.

An unfavourable result was presented for the Labiomental point which, despite a reduction in initial variability, was not sufficient to include the majority of markings within the 1% error limit adopted in this study, making it contraindicated for use in establishing facial patterns. For greater reliability in establishing vertical facial relationships, preference should be given to the other photoanthropometric points, which showed better results in this study.

An unfavourable result was presented for the Zygian point in relation to establishing facial patterns. However, its use for establishing horizontal facial dimensions was extremely favourable.

A Although it still requires adaptation and further study, the proposed photoanthropometric description can be applied to facial comparison analyses of images, providing a more categorical and scientific analysis, which are fundamental requirements for forensic analyses.

CHAPTER 8

Legal references

AKSU, M.; KAYA, D.; KOCADERELI, I. Reliability of reference distances used in photogrammetry. The Angle Orthodontist. 2010; 80(4): 660-677.

ALBENZ, G.O. Medicina legal e antropologia forense. Rio de Janeiro: Atheneu; 1988.

ALBERT, A.M.; RICANEK Jr., K.; PATTERSON E. A review of the literature on the aging adult skull and face: Implications for forensic science research and applications. Forensic Sci Int. 2007; 172: 1-9.

ALBUQUERQUE Jr., H.R.; ALMEIDA, M.H.C. Evaluation of the reproducibility error of cephalometric values applied in the Tweed-Merrifield philosophy, by computerised and conventional methods. Ortodontia. 1998; 31(3): 18-30.

ALDRIDGE, J. CCTV Operational Requirements Manual. Who will be the first to test your CCTV security or safety system? Police Scientific Development Branch (PSDB), 1994.

ALI, T.; VELDHUIS, R.N.J.; SPREEUWERS, L.J. Forensic Face Recognition: A Survey. Technical Report, Centre for Telematics and Information Technology University of Twente, Enschede: Netherlands, 2010.

ALLANSON, J.E. Objective techniques for craniofacial assessment: what are the choices? Am J Med Gen. 1997; 70: 1-5.

ALLANSON, J.E.; HENNEKAM, R.C.M.; MOOG, U.; SMEETS, E.E. Rett syndrome: A study of the face. Am J Med Genet. 2011; 155: 1563-1567.

ALLEN, R. Exact solutions to Bayesian and maximum likelihood problems in facial identification when population and error distributions are known. Forensic Sci Int. 2008; 179: 211- 218.

ALLEY, R. Social and Applied Aspects of Perceiving Faces. NJ: Lawrence Erlbaum Associates, Inc. 1998.

ALVES, A.P.P.P. Comparative analysis of facial anthropometry between parents of children with cleft lip and palate and individuals with no family history of clefts [Master's Thesis]. São Paulo: USP School of Dentistry; 2008.

ARRUDA, G.H.M. de; MORISSON, A.L. da C. Facial Recognition Examinations in the Federal Police. Proceedings of the International Conference on Forensic Sciences in Multimedia and Electronic Security. 2012. Brasília/DF, Brazil. p 78-85.

ASPRS. Manual of Photogrammetry. 6ª ed. American Society for Photogrammetry and Remote Sensing, 2013.

BATTAGEL, J.M. A comparative assessment of cephalometric errors. Eur J Orthod. 1993; 15: 305-314.

BENJAMIN, W. Charles Baudelaire: A Lyric poet in the Era of High Capitalism. London: NLB, 1983. p. 48.

BERTILLON, A. Signaletic instructions, including the Theory and Practice of Anthropometric Identification. Chicago: The Werner Company, 1896.

BISHARA, S.E.; CUMMINS, D.M.; JORGENSEN, G.J.; JAKOBSEN J.R. A computer assisted photogrammetric analysis of soft tissue changes after orthodontic treatment. Part I: Methodology and reliability. Am J Orthod Dentofacial Orthop, St. Louis. 1995; 107(6): 633639.

BISHARA, S.E.; JORGENSEN, G.J.; JAKOBSEN, J.R. Changes in facial dimensions assessed from lateral and frontal photographs. Part I - Methodology. Am J Orthod Dentofacial Orthop, St. Louis. 1998; 108(4): 389-393.

BRAZIL. Brazilian Penal Code (1941). Federative Republic of Brazil. Available at: <http://www.planalto.gov.br>. Accessed on 11 March 2014.

BRAZIL. Statute of the Child and Adolescent (1990). Federative Republic of Brazil. Federal Law No. 8069, of 13 July 1990. Available at:< http://www.planalto.gov.br>. Accessed on 11 March 2014.

BRUCE, V.; HENDERSON, Z.; BURTON, A. Factors affecting accuracy of verifying identities from CCTV images. Journal of Experimental Psychology. 2001; 7: 201-208.

BRUCE, V.; HENDERSON, Z.; GREENWOOD, K.; HANWOOD, P.; BURTON, A.M.; MILLER, P. Verification of face identities from images captured on video," Journal of Experimental Psychology. 2001; 5: 339-360.

BRUCE, V.; HENDERSON, Z.; NEWMAN, C.; BURTON, A.M. Matching identities of familiar and unfamiliar faces caught on CCTV images. J Exp Psychology. 2001; 7(3): 207-218.

BULUT, O.; SEVIM, A. The efficiency of anthropological examinations in forensic facial analysis. PBD. 2013; 15(1): 139-158.

BURTON, A. M.; MILLER, P.; BRUCE, V.; HANCOCK, P. J. B.; HENDERSON, Z. Human and automatic face recognition: a comparison across image formats. Vision Research. 2001; 41: 3185-3195.

BURTON, A.M.; WILSON, S.; COWAN, M.; BRUCE, V. Face recognition in poor-quality video: Evidence from security surveillance. Psychological Sci. 1999; 10(3): 243-248.

CARDOSO, M.A.; BERTOZ, F.A.; CAPELOZZA FILHO, L.; REIS, S.A.B. Cephalometric characteristics of the long face pattern. R Dental Press Ortodon Ortop Facial. 2005; 10(2): 2943.

CAROL, D.; BERKOWITZ, M.D. Child pornography: legal and medical considerations. Adv Pediatr. 2009; 56: 203-218.

CARROLL-MAYER, M.; FAIRWEATHER, B.; STAHL, B.C. CCTV Identity Management and Implications for Criminal Justice: some considerations. Surveillance & Society. 2008; 5(1): 33-50.

CATTANEO, C.; OBERTOVÁ, Z.; RATNAYAKE, M.; MARASCIUOLO, L.; TUTKUVIENE, J.; POPPA, P.; GIBELLI, D.; GABRIEL, P.; RITZ-TIMME, S. Can facial proportions taken from images be of use for ageing in cases of suspected child pornography? A pilot study. Int J Legal Med. 2012; 126: 139-144.

ÇELIKTUTAN, O.; ULUKAYA, S.; SANKUR, B. A comparative study of face landmarking techniques. EURASIP Journal on Image and Video Processing. 2013; 13: 1-27.

COHEN, A.M.; IP, H.H.; LINNEY, A.D. A preliminary study of computer recognition and identification of skeletal landmarks as a new method of cephalometric analysis. Br J Orthod. 1984; 11(3): 143-54.

COLOMBO, V.L.; MORO, A.; RECH, R.; VERONA, J.; COSTA, G.C. A. Frontal facial analysis at rest and during smiling in standardised photographs. Part I - Evaluation at rest. R Dental Press Ortodon Ortop Facial. 2004; 9(3): 47-58.

CUMMINS, D.M.; BISHARA, S.E.; JAKOBSEN, J.R. A computer assisted photogrammetric analysis of soft tissue changes after orthodontic treatment. Part II: Results. Am J Orthod Dentofacial Orthop, St. Louis. 1995; 108(1): 38-47.

DAVIS, J.P.; VALENTINE, T.; DAVIS, R.E. Computer assisted photo-anthropometric analyses of full-face and profile facial images. Forensic Sci Int. 2010; 200: 165-176.

DAVIS, J.P.; VALENTINE, T.; WILKINSON, C. Facial Image Comparison: Identification of the Living In: Craniofacial Identification, Wilkinson, C., and Rynn, C. Published by Cambridge University Press. Cambridge University Press 2012: 136-153.

DELIBERTI, J.H.; OLSON, D.P. Photogrammetric evaluation in clinical genetics: theoretical considerations and experimental results. Am J Med Genet 1991; 39: 161-6.

DEMAYO, C.; TORRES, M.; SINCO, A.; BONACHITA-SANGUILA, M. Geometric Morphometric Analyses of Facial Shape in Twins. The Internet Journal of Biological Anthropology. 2009; 4(1).

DIBEKLIOGLU, H. A Statistical Method for 2-D Facial Landmarking. IEEE Transactions on image processing. 2012; 21(2).

DOUGLAS, T.S. Image processing for craniofacial landmark identification and measurement: a review of photogrammetry and cephalometry. Computerised Medical Imaging and Graphics. 2004; 28: 401-409.

DOUGLAS, T.S.; MUTSVANGWA, T.E.M. A review of facial image analysis for delineation of the facial phenotype associated with fetal alcohol syndrome. Am J Med Genet. 2010; 152: 528-536.

EDMOND, G.; BIBER, K.; KEMP, R.; PORTER, G. Laws looking glass: expert identification evidence derived from photographic and video images. Curr Issues Crim Justice. 2009; 20(3): 337-377.

EKMAN, P.; FRIESEN, W.V. Unmasking the face: A guide to recognising emotions from facial expressions.

Ambridge, MA: Malor. 2003.

ENLOW, D.H. Facial Growth. 3ª ed. Philadelphia: W.B. Saunders Company; 1990.

ENLOW, D.H.; HANS, M.G. Essentials of facial growth. Philadelphia: W.B. Saunders Company; 1996.

ENLOW, D.H.; POSTON, W.R.; BAKOR, S.F. Facial growth. 3ª ed. Artes Médicas; 1993.

FABRIS, A. Attendance certificates: photography as a scientific tool. Locus: Journal of History. Juiz de Fora. 2002; 8(1).

FABRIS, A. Identidades virtuais: uma leitura do retrato fotográfico. Belo Horizonte: UFMG, 2004. p40.

FISWIG. FACIAL IDENTIFICATION SCIENTIFIC WORKING GROUP. Guidelines for Facial Comparison Methods. 2012. Available at: http://www.fiswg.org/FISWG_GuidelinesforFacialComparisonMethods_v1.0_2012_02_02 .pdf. [Accessed 10 Mar 2014].

FACIAL IDENTIFICATION SCIENTIFIC WORKING GROUP (FISWIG). Capture and Equipment Assessment for FRSystems. 2011. Available at: http://www.fiswg.org/FISWG_CaptureAndEquipmentAssessmentForFRSystems_v1.0_20 11_05_05.pdf. [Accessed 10 Mar 2014].

FARKAS, G.L.; BRYSON, W.; KLOTZ, J. Is photogrammetry of the face reliable? Plast Reconstr Surg. 1980; 66: 346-355.

FARKAS, J.G.; DEUTSCH, C.K. Anthropometric Determination of Craniofacial Morphology. American Journal of Medical Genetics. 1996; 65: 1-4.

FARKAS, L.G. Accuracy of Anthropometric Measurements: Past, Present, and Future. Cleft Palate-Craniovacial Journal. 1996; 33: 10-22.

FARKAS, L.G. Anthropometry of the Head and Face, 2nd ed. New York: Raven Press. 1994: 2125.

FARKAS, L.G.; MUNRO, I.R. Anthropometric Facial Proportions in Medicine. Charles C Thomas, Springfield, Illinois, USA, 1987.

FERRARA, M.; FRANCO, A.; MALTONI, D. Evaluating systems assessing face-image compliance with ICAO/ISO standards. *BIOID, volume 5372 of Lecture Notes in Computer Science.* Springer-Verlag Berlin Heidelberg. 2008: 191-199.

FERRARO, M.M.; CASEY, E.; MCGRATH, M. Investigating child exploitation and pornography: the internet, the law and forensic science. Academic: New York, 2004.

FORSYTH, D.B.; DAVIS, D.N. Assessment of an automated cephalometric analysis system. Eur J Orthod. 1996; 18(5): 471-8.

GEORGE, R.M. Facial Geometry: Graphic Facial Analysis for Forensic Artists. Springfield: Charles C Thomas Publisher LTD; 2007.

GERRARD, G.; PARKINS, G.; CUNNINGHAM, I.; JONES, W.; HILL, S.; DOUGLAS, S. National CCTV Strategy. London: Home Office, 2007.

GIL, C.T.L. DE A.; GROSSI, A.T.R.; SILVA, F.P.L. da; MALTAGLIATI, L.A. Determination and localisation of the OPI point in lateral cephalometric radiographs. Odonto - Revista de Odontologia da Metodista. Editora da Universidade Metodista. 2004; 12(23): 63-73.

GILL, M.; SPRIGGS, A. Assessing the impact of CCTV. Home Office Research Study 292. Home Office Research, Development and Statistics Directorate, 2005. Available at: http://www.homeoffice.gov.uk/rds/pdfs05/hors292.pdf> [Accessed 20 Mar 2014].

GINZBURG, C. Myths, emblems, signs: morphology and history. São Paulo: Companhia das Letras, 1989. p. 173.

GOLDSTEIN, A.J.; HARMON, L.D.; LESK, A.B. Identification of human faces. 1971; 59(5): 748-760.

GOOLD, B. Privacy Rights and Public Spaces: CCTV and the Problem of the 'Unobservable Observer'.

Criminal Justice Ethics. 2002; 21(1).

GOULD, S.J. The Mismeasure of Man. New York: W.W. Norton & Company.1981.

GUNNING, T. The portrait of the human body: photography, detectives and the beginnings of cinema. In: CHARNEY, L., SCHWARTZ, V. O cinema e invenção da vida moderna. 2ª ed. São Paulo: Cosac & Naify. 2004: 43-48.

GUYOT, L.; DUBUC, M.; RICHARD, O.; PHILIP, N.; DUTOUR, O. Comparison between direct clinical and digital photogrammetric measurements in patients with 22q11 microdeletion. Int J Oral Maxillofac Surg. 2003; 32(3): 246-52.

GUYURON, B. Precision rhinoplasty. Part I: the role of life-size photographs and soft tissue cephalometric analysis. Plast Reconstr Surg. 1988; 81: 489-99.

HALBERSTEIN, R.A. The application of anthropometric indices in forensic photography: three case studies. J Forensic Sci. 2001; 46(6): 1438-41.

HALL, J.G.; GRIPP, K.W.; SLAVOTINEK, A.M. Handbook of physical measurements. 2ª ed. USA: Oxford University Press; 2006.

HARPER, B.; LATTO, R. Cyclopean vision, size estimation, and presence in orthostereoscopic images. Presence. 2001; 10(3): 312-330.

HENNEBERG, M.; SIMPSON, E.; STEPHAN, C. Human Face in Biological Anthropology: Craniometry, Evolution and Forensic Identification. In: The human face: Measurement and Meaning. Mary Katsikitis. Boston: Kluwer Academic Publishers. 2003: 29-48.

HENNESSY, R.J.; MOSS, J.P. Facial growth: separating shape from size. European Journal of Orthodontics. 2001; 23: 275-285.

HENRIQUES, A.P.; NAVES, T. de O.; BICALHO, G.C.; VIDAL, F. de B.; BORGES, D.L. A proposal for a tool forensic investigation in images. Proceedings of the International Conference on Multimedia and

Electronic Security Forensic Sciences . Brasília/DF, Brazil. 2012: 74-77.

HARRELL, T.W.M. A invenção da fotografia in: Manual de Fotografia. 2002. p. 4-15.

HESS, E. Facial Recognition: A Valuable Tool for Law Enforcement. Forensic Magazine. 2010; 7(5).

HOFER, M.; MARANA, A.N. Dental biometrics: Human Identification based on dental work information. Diploma Thesis. 2007.

HOUAISS, A. Novo Dicionário Houaiss da Língua Portuguesa. Antônio Houaiss Institute. Publisher: Editora Objetiva, 2009.

ICAO. International Civil Aviation Organisation. Biometrics Deployment of Machine Readable Travel Documents. ICAO TAG MRTD/NTWG, 2004.

ICAO. International Civil Aviation Organisation. Doc 9303: Machine Readable Travel Documents. 6ª ed. Part 1: Machine Readable Passports. Volume 1: Passports with Machine Readable Data Stored in Optical Character Recognition Format, 2006.

ÍÇCAN, M.Y. Introduction to techniques for photographic comparison: potentials and problems. In M. Y. I§can and R. P. Helmer, Forensic Analysis of the Skull: Craniofacial Analysis, Reconstruction, and Identification. New York: Wiley-Liss. 1993: 57-70.

ÍÇCAN, M.Y.; LOTH, S.R. Photo Image Identification. In Siegel, J.A., Saukko, P.J., Knupfer, G.C. Encyclopaedia of Forensic Sciences. London: Academic Press. 2000: 795-807.

ISO/IEC 19794-5. Information technology: Biometric data interchange formats. 2ª ed. Part 5: Face image data, 2011.

IVERSEN, E.; SHIBATA, Y. Canon and proportions in Egyptian art. 2ª ed. Warminster: Aris and Phillips, 1975.

JAIN, A.K.; BRENDAN, K.; UNSANG, P.A.R.K. Face Matching and Retrieval in Forensics Applications. In:

Multimedia in Forensics, Security, and Intelligence. Michigan State University. IEEE Computer Society. 2012: 2-10.

JURMAIN, R.; KILGORE, L.; TREVANTHAN, W. Essentials of Physical Anthropology, Seventh Edition. Wadsworth, Cengage Learning; 2009.

KAU, C.H.; RICHMOND, S.; INCRAPERA, A.; ENGLISH, J.; XIA, J.J. Three-dimensional surface acquisition systems for the study of facial morphology and their application to maxillofacial surgery. Int J Med Robot Comput Assist Surg. 2007; 3: 97-110.

KERRY, S.; HOWITT, D. Sex offenders and the internet. Wiley: New York, 2007.

KEVAL, H.U.; SASSE, M.A. Can we ID from CCTV: image quality in digital CCTV and face identification performance. In: Agaian, S.S., Jassim, S.A., (eds.) Mobile multimedia/image processing, security, and applications. 2008: K9820 - K9820.

KLEINBERG, K.F.; PHARM, B.; VANESIZ, P.; BURTON, M.A. Failure of anthropometry as a facial identification technique using high quality photographs, J. Forensic Sci. 2007; 52(4): 779-783.

KLEINBERG, K.F. Facial anthropometry as an evidential tool in forensic image comparison. PhD thesis. University of Glasgow. 2008.

KOLAR, J.C.; SALTER, E.M. Craniofacial anthropometry: practical measurement of the head and face for clinical, surgical, and research use. Springfield: Charles C Thomas Publisher LTD; 1997.

KRISHAN, K.; KANCHAN, T. Anthropometric and Anthroposcopic Analysis of Face in Forensic Identification-Some Essential. Medico-Legal Considerations Update. 2012; 12(1).

KUNJUR, J.; SABESAN, T.; ILANKOVAN, V. Anthropometric analysis of eyebrows and eyelids: An interracial study. Brit J Oral Maxillofac Surg. 2006; 44: 89-93.

LAU, P.; COOKE, M.S.; HÀGG, U. Effects of training and experience on cephalometric measurement errors on surgical patients. J Adult Orthod. 1997; 12(3): 204-213.

LEE, W.; WILKINSON, C.; MEMON, A.; HOUSTON, K. Matching Unfamiliar Faces from Poor Quality Closed-Circuit Television (CCTV) Footage. 2009; 1(1).

LI, J.; CHU, S.; PAN, J.; JAIN, L.C. Multiple Viewpoints Based Overview for Face Recognition. Journal of Information Hiding and Multimedia Signal Processing. 2012; 3(4): 352-369.

LUZ, F.A.O. Real object dimensioning through image capture in digital systems. [Master's dissertation]. Federal University of Paraná-UFPR. Curitiba, 2011.

MACHADO, C.E.P.; FILHO, E.G. de L.; ARRUDA, G.H.M. de.; REIS, P.M.G.I. Facial Recognition. Workbook for the VI Facial Recognition Course. Ministry of Justice. Federal Police Department, 2014.

MARTIN, R.; SALLER K. Lehrbuch der Anthropologie Band 1, 3rd edn. In: G. Fisher, Stuttgart, 1957.

MARTINS, L.P.; PINTO, A.S.; MARTINS, J.C.R.; MENDES, A.J.D. Reproducibility error of Steiner and Ricketts cephalometric analysis measurements, by conventional and computerised methods. Rev Ortodontia. 1995; 28(1): 04-17.

McCAHILL, M.; NORRIS, C. Estimating the extent, sophistication and legality of CCTV in London. In M. Gill, CCTV. Leicester: Perpetuity Press, 2003.

MIKHAIL, E.; ACKERMAN, F. Observations and Least Squares. University Press of America, 1976. 64 p.

MITCHELL, H.L.; NEWTON, I. Medical photogrammetric measurement: overview and prospects. ISPRS J Photogrammetry Remote Sensing. 2002; 56(5-6): 286-94.

MORECROFT, L.; FIELLER, N.R.J.; EVISON, M.P. Investigation of Anthropometric Landmarking in 2D. In: Computer-Aided Forensic Facial Comparison. CRC Press: Boca Raton, FL. 2010: 71-87.

MORETON, R.; MORLEY, J. Investigation into the use of photoanthropometry in facial image comparison. Forensic Sci Int. 2011; 212(1): 231-237.

MUTSVANGWA, T.; DOUGLAS, T.S. Morphometric analysis of facial landmark data to characterise the facial phenotype associated with fetal alcohol syndrome. J Anat. 2007; 210: 209-220.

NASA. Anthropometric Source Book. National Aeronautics and Space Administration. Government Printing Office: Washington, D.C. 1978; 1.

NIST. National Institute of Standards and Technology. Facial Recognition Vendor Test, 2006. Available at: http://face.nist.gov/. [Accessed 23 Jan 2014].

NORRIS, C.; McCAHILL, M.; WOOD, D. The growth of CCTV: a global perspective on the international diffusion of video surveillance in publicly accessible space. Surveillance and Society. Editorial. 2004: 2(2/3): 110-135.

PATIAS, P. ISPRS Journal of Photogrammetry & Remote Sensing. 2002; 56: 295-310.

PEREIRA, C.B.; ALVIM, M.C.D.M.E. Manual for craniometric and cranioscopic studies. University City: Federal University of Santa Maria, 1979. 125 p.

PERINI, T.A.; OLIVEIRA, G.L. de; ORNELLAS, J. dos S.; OLIVEIRA, F.P. de. Technical error of measurement in anthropometry. Rev Bras Med Esporte. 2005; 11: (1).

PETROSKI, E.L. Development and validation of generalised equations for estimating body density in adults. [Doctoral Thesis]. Santa Maria, RS: UFSM, 1995.

PHAM, A.M.; TOLLEFSON, T.T. Objective Facial Photograph Analysis Using Imaging Software. Facial Plast Surg Clin N Am. 2010; 18: 341-349.

PHELINE, C. L'image accusatrice, Les Cahiers de la Photographie, Paris, n. 17, 1985.

PHILLIPS, P.J.; SCRUGGS, W.T.; O'TOOLE, A. J. FRVT 2006 and ICE 2006: Large-scale Results. National Institute of Standards and Technology. NISTIR 7408, 2007. Available at: http://iris.nist.gov [Accessed 10 Dec 2013].

PORTER, G.; DORAN, G. An anatomical and photographic technique for forensic facial identification. Forensic Sci Int. 2000; 114(2): 97-105.

PROFFIT, W.R.; ACKERMAN, J.L. Diagnosis and planning of orthodontic treatment. In: Graber TM Vanarsdall RL. Orthodontics: current principles and techniques. 2ª ed. Rio de Janeiro: Guanabara Koogan; 1996. p.3-87.

PURKAIT, R. Anthropometric landmarks: How reliable are they? Anthropometric landmarks. Med Leg Update. 2004;4(4):133-40.

RAI, B.; KAUR, J. Craniofacial Identification in: Legal Odontology. Evidence-based Berlin Heidelberg: Springer-Verlag, 2013, p.66.

RAKOSI, T. An atlas of ceophalometric radiography. London: Wolfe Medical Publications; 1982.

RAMANATHAN, N.; CHELLAPPA, R. Modelling age progression in young faces. University of Maryland: College Park, 2006.

RAS, F.; HABETS, L.L.M.H.; VAN GINKEL, F.C.; PRAHL-ANDERSEN, B. Quantification of facial morphology using stereophotogrammetry-demonstration of a new concept. J Dent. 1996; 24(5): 369-74.

REN, C.; DAI, D. Incremental learning of bidirectional principal components for face recognition. Pattern Recognition. 2010; 43(1): 318-330.

RHODES, G. The evolutionary psychology of facial beauty. Annu Rev Psychol. 2006; 57: 199226.

RHODES, G.; PROFFITT, F.; GRADY, J.M.; SUMICH, A. Facial symmetry and the perception of beauty. Psvchonomic Bulletin & Review. 1998; 5(4): 659-669.

RICHARDSON, A. A comparison of traditional and computerised methods of cephalometric analysis. Eur J Orthod. 1981; 3: 15-20.

ROELOFSE, M.; STEYN, M.; BECKER, P. Photo identification: Facial metrical and morphological features in South African males. Forensic Sci Int. 2008; 177: 168-175.

SAMAIN, E. When photography (already) made anthropologists dream. Revista de Antropologia. São Paulo, USP. 2001; 44(2): 89-126.

SAMAL, A.; IYENGAR, P. Automatic recognition and analysis of human faces and facial expressions: a survey. Pattern Recognit. 1992; 25(1): 65-77.

SANTOS, R.; FURJÃO, C. Anthropometry. University of Évora - Postgraduate Course: Higher Technician in HST. February 2003.

SCORSATO, H. The use of photography in identification processes and the Bertillon method - 19th century. Estudios Historicos, Uruguay. 2012; 9.

SFORZA, C.; GRANDI, G.; CATTI, F.; TOMMASI, D. Age- and sex-related changes in the soft tissues of the orbital region. Forensic Sci Int. 2009; 185(8): 115.e1-115.e8.

SHELDON, W.H.; STEVENS, S.S.; TUCKER, W.B. The varieties of human physique. Oxford, England: Harper. 1940; 12: 347 pp.

SHI, J.; SAMAI, A.; MARX, D. How effective are landmarks and their geometry for face recognition? Computer vision and image understanding. 2006; 102(2): 117-133.

SINHA, P. Symmetry sensing through computer vision and a facial recognition system. Forensic Science International. 1996; 77: 27-36.

SOBRAL, F. Perfil Morfológico e Prestação Desportiva: Estudo Antropométrico do Desportista de Alto Nível de Rendimento. Lisbon: Portugal, 1985.

STAVRIANOS, C.; PAPADOPOULOS, C.; PANTELIDOU, O.; EMMANOUIL, J.; PENTALOTIS, N.; TATSIS, D. The use of photoanthropometry in facial mapping. Research Journal of Medical Sciences. 2012; 6(4): 166-169.

STEELE, J. Face to face. Analysis and Comparison of Facial Features to authenticate identities of people in photographs. 2nd Ed. United States of America (Washington): Joelle Steele Interprises, 2013.

STEVENS, R.; CALHOUN, K.; QUINN, F.B. Facial Analysis. University of Texas Medical Branch. Dept of Otolaryngology. University of Texas Medical Branch. 1997. Available at:

http://www.utmb.edu/otoref/grnds/ZX/facial2.html [Accessed 6 Nov 2013].

STONEY, D.A. What made us ever think we could individualise using statistics? JFSS. 1991; 31(2): 197-99.

STRAUSS, R.A.; WEIS, B.D.; LINDAUER, S.J.; REBELLATO, J.; ISAACSON, R.J. Variability of facial photographs for use in treatment planning for orthodontics and orthognathic surgery. Int J Adult Orthod Orthognath Surg, Lombard. 1997; 12(3): 197-203.

SWGIT. SCIENTIFIC WORKING GROUP ON IMAGING TECHNOLOGY (2004), Recommendations and Guidelines for Using Closed-Circuit Television Security Systems in

Commercial Institutions. Available at: http://www.theiai.org/guidelines/swgit/index.php> [Accessed 20 Feb 2014].

TAYLOR, D.; MYERS, W.C.; ROBBINS, L.; BARNARD, G.W. An anthropometric study of paedophiles and rapists. J Forensic Sci. 1993; 38(4): 765-768.

TAYLOR, K. Forensic Art and Illustration. Boca Ratan: CRC Press; 2001.

VALE, F.J.F. do. Aesthetic analysis of the face of the Portuguese population based on the natural position of the head. Faculty of Medicine, University of Coimbra, 2004 [Master's dissertation].

VEGTER, F.; HAGE, J.J. Clinical Anthropometry and Canons of the Face in Historical Perspective. plastic and reconstructive surgery. 2000; 106: 1090-1096.

VLAHOS, J. Surveillance Society: New High-Tech Cameras Are Watching You. Popular Mechanics. 2009. Available at: www.popularmechanics.com/ technology/military/4236865 [Accessed 3 January 2014].

WIERZBICKI, S.L. Reproducibility of cephalometric points and their importance in interpreting the A-Nperp magnitude of McNamara's analysis - A review study [Specialisation Monograph]. Curitiba: Universidade Tuiuti do Paraná; 2011.

WILKINSON, C. Forensic Facial Reconstruction. Cambridge: Cambridge University Press; 2008.

WILKINSON, C.; EVANS, R. Are facial image analysis experts any better than the general public at identifying individuals from CCTV images? Sci Justice. 2009; 49(3): 191-196.

YOSHINO, M.; NOGUCHI, K.; ATSUCHI, M.; KUBOTA, S.; IMAIZUMI, K.; THOMAS, C.D.; CLEMENT, J.G. Individual identification of disguised faces by morphometrical matching. Forensic Sci Int. 2002;127:97-103.

ZAR, J. H. Biostatistical analysis. 4ª ed. New Jersey: Prentice Hall, 1999.

ZIMBLER, M.S.; HAM, J. Aesthetic Facial Analysis. Otolaryngology-Head and Neck Surgery, Cummings Editor, 4ª ed, 2005. Mosby.

GLOSSARY

Contralateral - On the opposite side.

Hemiface - Each half of the face.

Ipsilateral or Homolateral - On the same side.

Neurocranium - Part of the skeleton of the head that forms the cranial cavity and houses the encephalon.

Smart card - A plastic ***card*** with a magnetic stripe that is used as identification to access networks, computers and devices.

Viscerocranium - Part of the skeleton of the head that corresponds to the face.

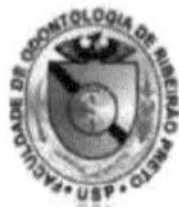

SERVIÇO PÚBLICO FEDERAL
MINISTÉRIO DA JUSTIÇA
DEPARTAMENTO DE POLÍCIA FEDERAL

UNIVERSIDADE DE SÃO PAULO
FACULDADE DE ODONTOLOGIA DE RIBEIRÃO PRETO
PROGRAMA DE REABILITAÇÃO ORAL

MANUAL DE MARCAÇÃO DE PONTOS FOTOANTROPOMÉTRICOS SOBRE IMAGENS FACIAIS EM NORMA FRONTAL COM USO DO SOFTWARE SMVFACE

Autores:
Marta Regina Pinheiro Flores*
Carlos Eduardo Palhares Machado**
Marco Aurelio Guimarães***
Ricardo Henrique Alves da Silva****

* Pós-graduanda nível Mestrado da Faculdade de Odontologia de Ribeirão Preto, Universidade de São Paulo (FORP/USP)
** Pós-graduando nível Doutorado da Faculdade de Medicina de Ribeirão Preto, Universidade de São Paulo (FMRP/USP)
*** Professor Doutor da Faculdade de Medicina de Ribeirão Preto, Universidade de São Paulo (FMRP/USP)
**** Professor Doutor da Faculdade de Odontologia de Ribeirão Preto, Universidade de São Paulo (FORP/USP)

APRESENTAÇÃO INICIAL

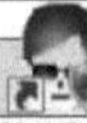

SMVFace

Ao abrir o programa SMVFace, aparecerá uma tela contendo um diagrama à esquerda com vários pontos faciais numerados, sendo que os pontos de número **1**, **1e**, **2** e **2e** aparecem em vermelho e os demais, em preto. À direita da tela, é possível visualizar uma janela em preto, onde as fotografias serão inseridas e visualizadas (Figura 1).

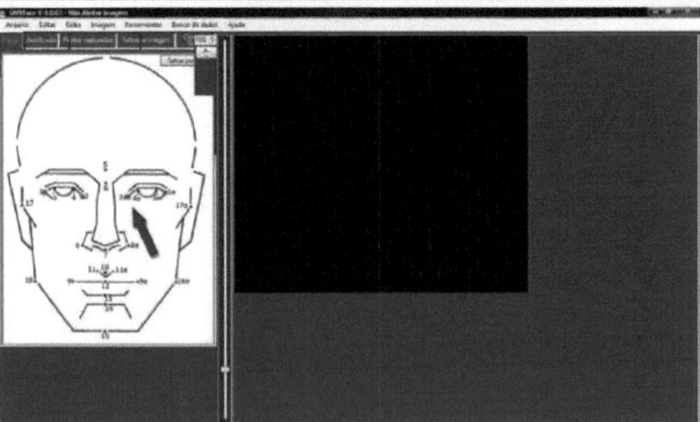

Figura 1

ORIENTAÇÕES - ABRIR IMAGEM

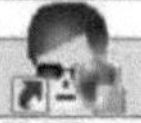

SMVFace

Para abrir uma imagem, clique no comando "**Arquivo**" da barra de menu e depois em "**Abrir imagem**" (Figura 2).

Selecionar a imagem predeterminada. A imagem aparecerá no lado direito da tela juntamente com uma linha horizontal verde e uma vertical azul (Figura 3). Estas serão utilizadas como guia na determinação dos pontos.

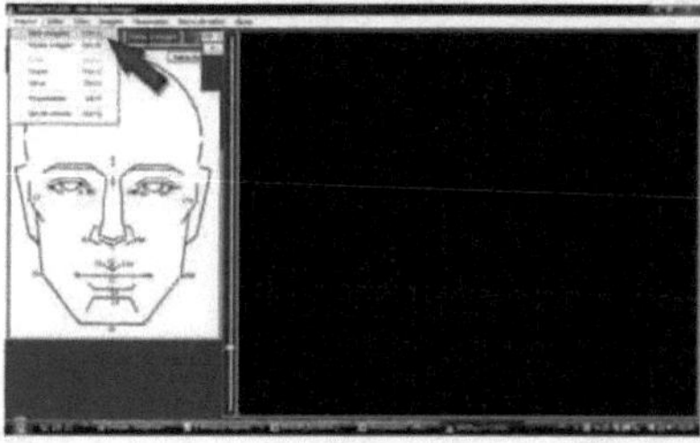

Figura 2

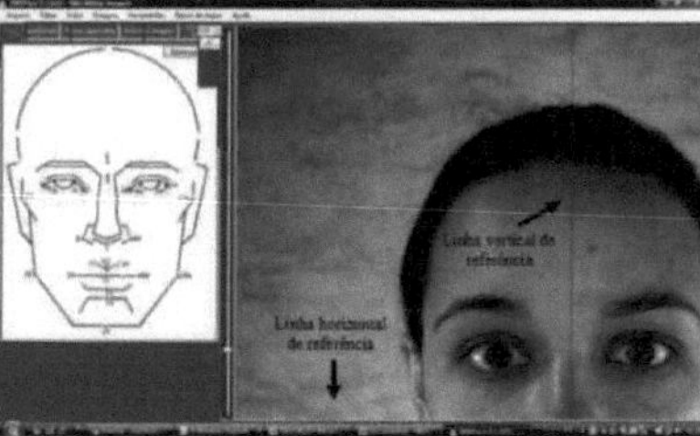

Figura 3

ORIENTAÇÕES - MARCAÇÃO DO PONTO

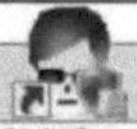

SMVFace

Para marcar um ponto facial, primeiramente selecione o ponto desejado no layout esquerdo da tela. Os pontos liberados para a marcação estão em vermelho (Figura 4). Após a seleção do ponto, o mesmo mudará de cor (tornando-se amarelo) e ficará piscando.

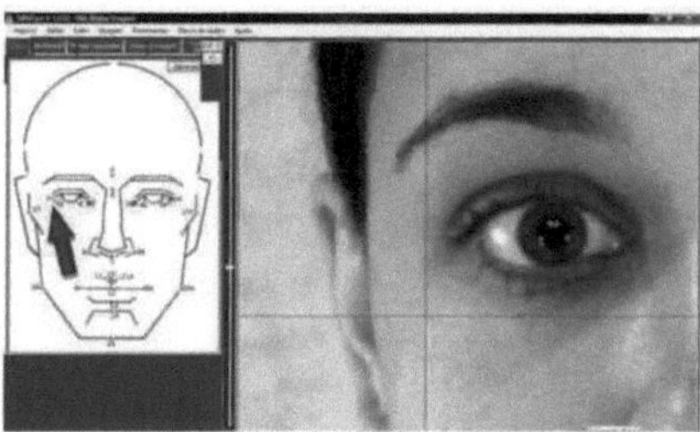

Figura 4

ORIENTAÇÕES - MARCAÇÃO DO PONTO

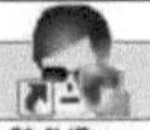

Para determinar o ponto escolhido na imagem, posicione o marcador no local desejado e clique com o botão esquerdo do mouse. Posicione o marcador na fotografia utilizando as linhas guia (Figura 5).

O ponto marcado inicialmente na foto é amarelo e, estando nessa condição, permite a utilização da tecla "**Ctrl + setas**" para corrigir pequenos erros de posicionamento, ou ainda por meio do cursor no canto superior esquerdo da fotografia.

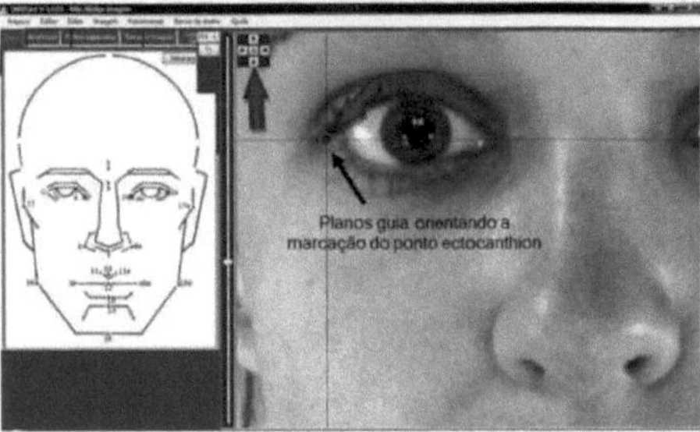

Figura 5

ORIENTAÇÕES - DETERMINAÇÃO DO PONTO

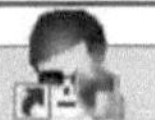

Caso esteja certo de sua marcação, aperte a tecla "**Enter**" para a determinação final do ponto. O ponto selecionado na foto ficará vermelho e o ponto no layout esquerdo ficará verde, assinalando que o mesmo já foi determinado (Figura 6). Após o posicionamento de cada ponto e antes de apertar "**Enter**", é aconselhado reduzir a ampliação da imagem a fim de verificar o adequado posicionamento do ponto (Figura 7).

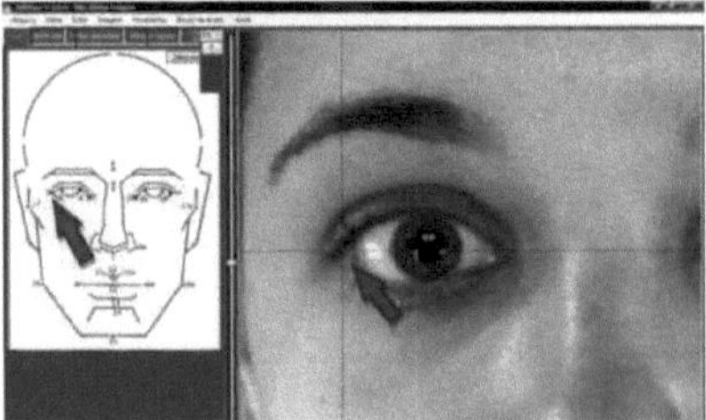

Figura 6

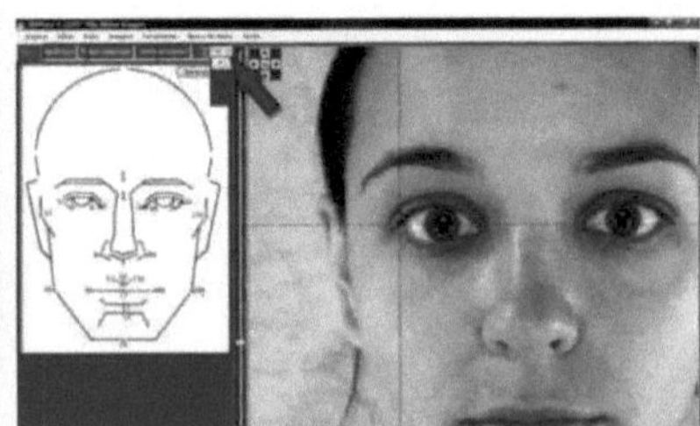

Figura 7

ORIENTAÇÕES

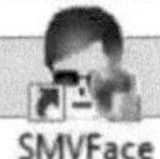

Para refazer um ponto já marcado, clique no ícone "**Editar**" e depois em "**Desfazer**" ou então, selecione novamente o ponto no layout esquerdo e marque novamente na posição correta (Figura 8).

Ao final da marcação dos 22 pontos cefalométricos de cada fotografia, clique em "**Salvar pontos**" (Figura 9).

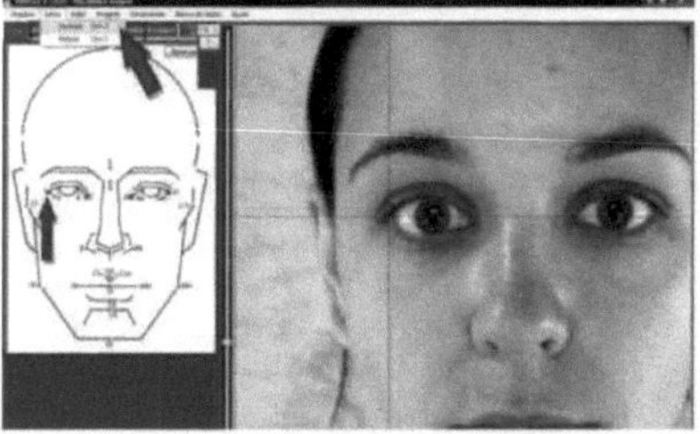

Figura 8

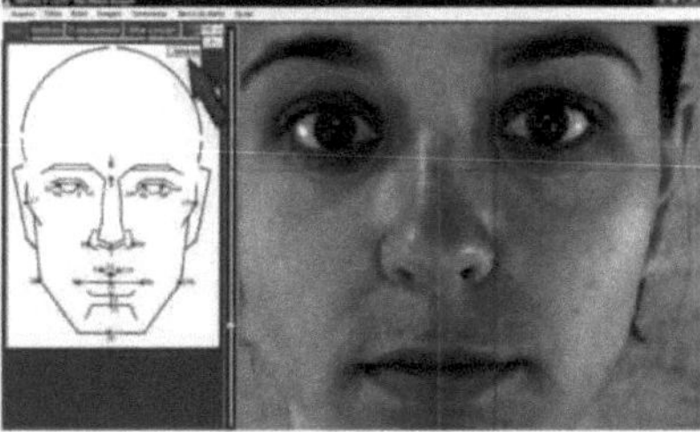

Figura 9

1. ECTOCANTHION

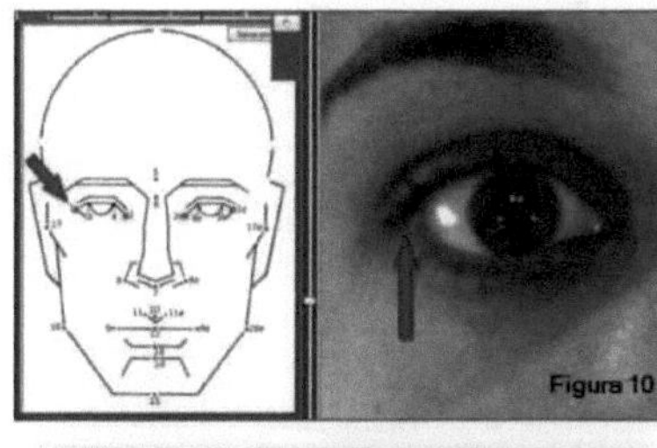

Figura 10

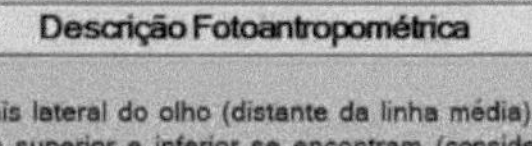

Descrição Fotoantropométrica

Ponto mais lateral do olho (distante da linha média), onde as pálpebras superior e inferior se encontram (considerar como referência a região de encontro das linhas de implantação dos cílios superiores e inferiores e não a região de ângulo interno, próxima à parte branca do olho).

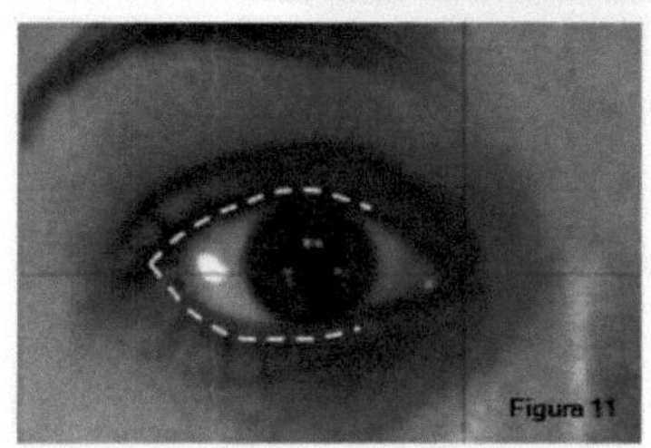

Figura 11

Procedimentos para a marcação do ponto

Selecionar o ponto número 1 no diagrama facial (seta Fig. 10) e dar zoom na imagem até o enquadramento do olho analisado, se a resolução permitir. Deverão ser utilizadas as linhas de referência para a marcação do ponto, deslocando primeiramente a **linha vertical** do lado lateral para medial da face e, posteriormente, a **linha horizontal** de baixo para cima até posiciona-las na região de encontro das pálpebras superior e inferior (observar linha pontilhada na Fig. 11). O ectocanthion deverá ser marcado na região de interseção entre as duas linhas de referência. Se o cílio estiver cobrindo a região, deverá ser marcada a região estimada. Seguir o mesmo procedimento para marcação do ponto contralateral (**1e**).

2. ENDOCANTHION

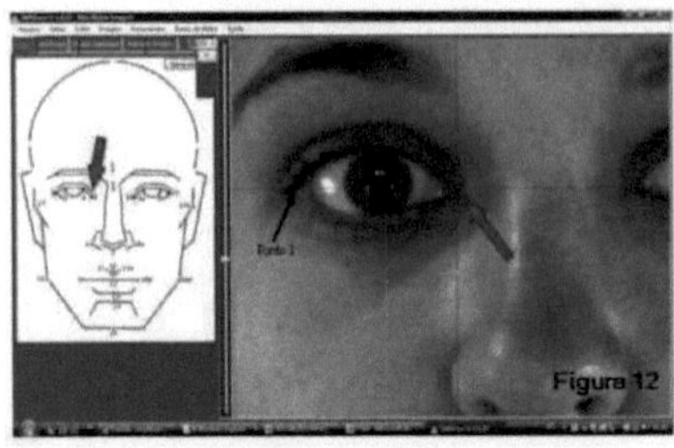

Figura 12

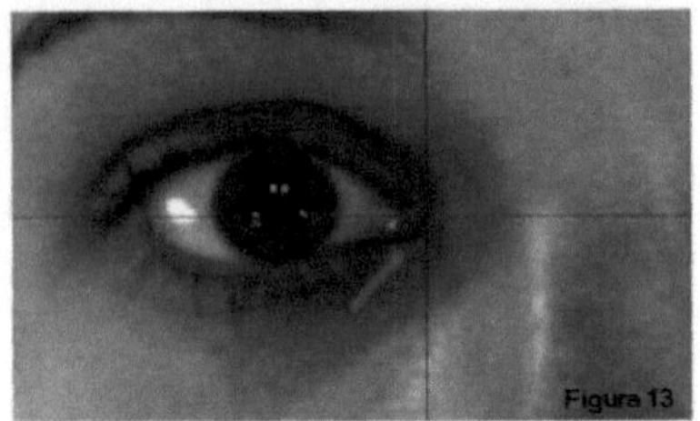

Figura 13

Descrição Fotoantropométrica

Ponto mais interno do olho (próximo da linha média), onde as pálpebras superior e inferior se encontram (considerar como referência a região mais medial de encontro das linhas de implantação dos cílios superiores e inferiores e não a região de ângulo interno, próxima à carúncula lacrimal).

Procedimentos para a marcação do ponto

Selecionar o ponto número 2 no diagrama facial (seta Fig. 12) e dar zoom na imagem até o enquadramento do olho analisado, se a resolução permitir. Deverão ser utilizadas as linhas de referência para a marcação do ponto, deslocando primeiramente a **linha vertical** do lado medial para lateral da face e, posteriormente, a **linha horizontal** de baixo para cima até posiciona-las na região de encontro das pálpebras superior e inferior (Fig. 13). O endocanthion deverá ser marcado na região de interseção entre as duas linhas de referência. Seguir o mesmo procedimento para marcação do ponto contralateral (**2e**).

OBSERVAÇÃO

Após a determinação dos pontos **1**, **1e**, **2** e **2e** aparecerá uma linha média (linha média orbital) em um tom mais claro do que as linhas de referência vertical e horizontal (Figura 14).

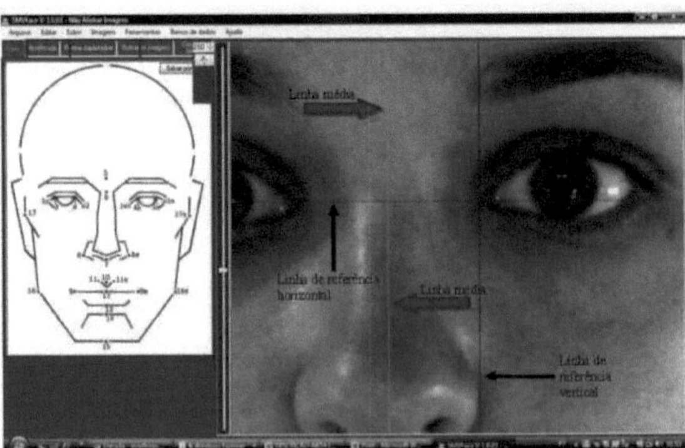

Figura 14

OBSERVAÇÃO

Para ativar e desativar a linha média orbital, clique em "**Exibir**" e depois em "**Linha média**" (Figura 15).

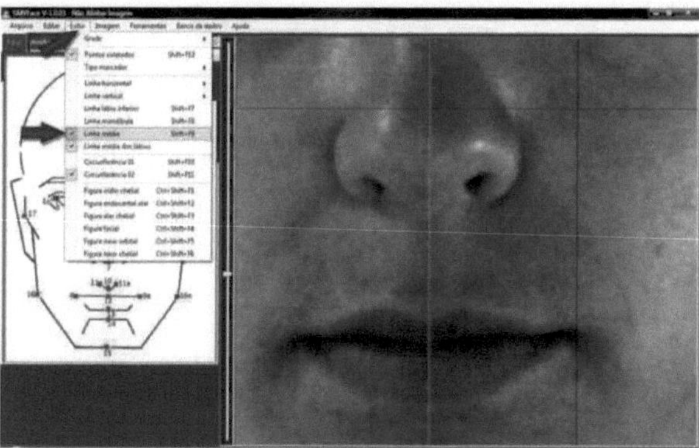

Figura 15

OBSERVAÇÃO

Para ativar e desativar as linhas verticais e horizontais de referência, clique em "**Exibir**" e depois selecione as linhas de interesse dentro do ícone "**Linha vertical**" (Figura 16) e "**Linha horizontal**" (Figura 17).

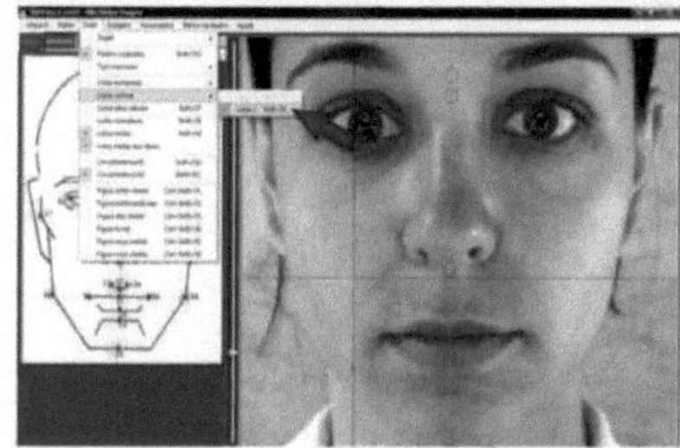

Figura 16

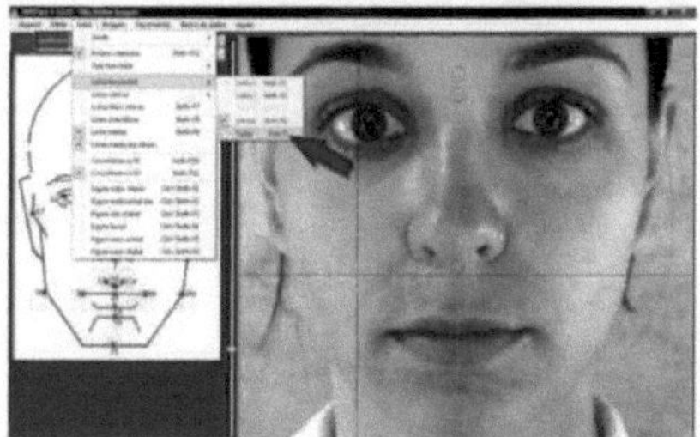

Figura 17

3. IRÍDIO LATERAL

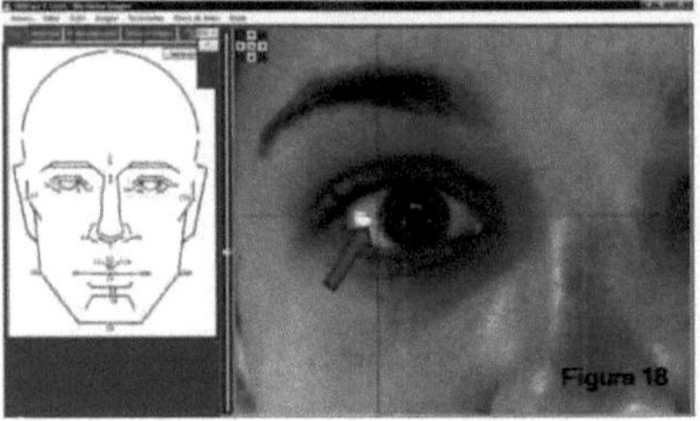
Figura 18

Descrição Fotoantropométrica

Ponto mais lateral da circunferência colorida do olho (olho direito ou esquerdo). **Onde a circunferência possui o maior diâmetro.** É o ponto de tangência da linha de referência vertical em relação a circunferência mais externa e lateral da íris.

Procedimentos para a marcação do ponto

Selecionar o ponto número 3 no diagrama facial e dar zoom na imagem até o enquadramento do olho analisado, se a resolução permitir. Deverão ser utilizadas as linhas de referência para a marcação do ponto, deslocando primeiramente a **linha vertical** do lado lateral para medial da face e, posteriormente, a **linha horizontal** de baixo para cima até posiciona-las na região de maior circunferência da íris. O irídio lateral deverá ser marcado na região de interseção entre elas (vide imagem ao lado). Seguir o mesmo procedimento para marcação do ponto contralateral (**3e**).

4. IRÍDIO MEDIAL

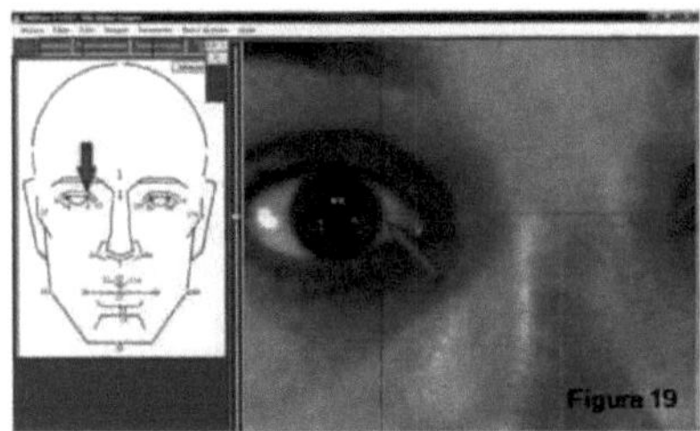
Figura 19

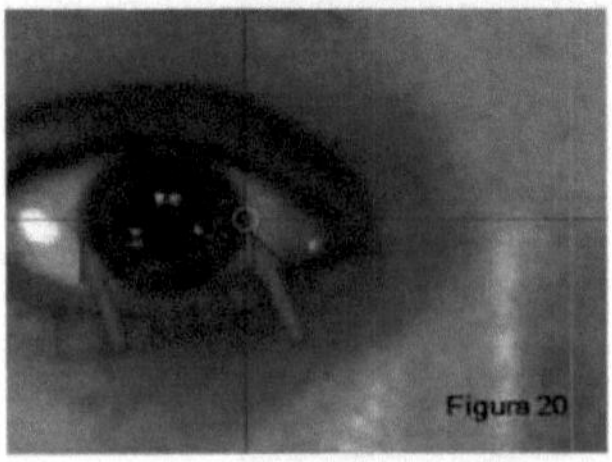

Figura 20

Descrição Fotoantropométrica

Ponto mais medial da circunferência colorida do olho (olho direito ou esquerdo). É o ponto de tangência da linha de referência vertical em relação à circunferência mais externa e medial da íris.

Procedimentos para a marcação do ponto

Selecionar o ponto número 4 no diagrama facial (seta vermelha Fig. 19) e dar zoom na imagem até o enquadramento do olho analisado, se a resolução permitir. A **linha horizontal** de referência deverá ser posicionada na mesma posição utilizada para a determinação do ponto 3, ou seja, a linha horizontal de referência deve passar por ambos os pontos irídios do mesmo lado facial em análise, mesmo que, aparentemente, não corresponda à maior circunferência da íris medialmente (Fig. 20). Deslocar a **linha vertical** do lado medial para lateral da face até que a mesma tangencie a circunferência da íris. O irídio medial deverá ser marcado na região de interseção entre as linhas de referência. Seguir o mesmo procedimento para marcação do ponto contralateral (**4e**).

OBSERVAÇÃO

Os pontos marcados em etapa anterior permanecem assinalados, tanto na fotografia como no diagrama à esquerda. No exemplo, os pontos **1** e **2** aparecem assinalados durante a marcação do ponto **3** (Figura 21).

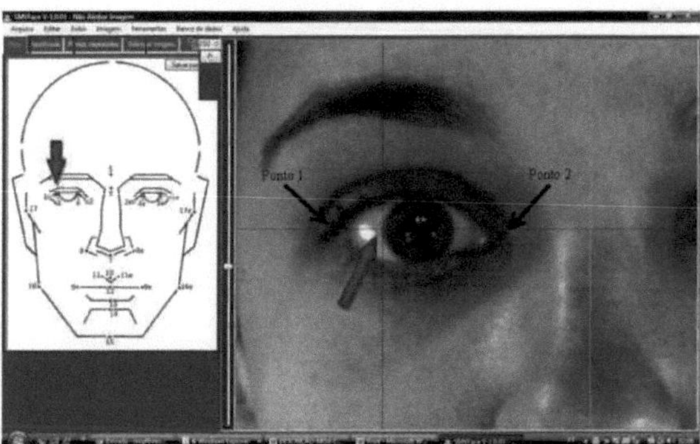

Figura 21

OBSERVAÇÃO

Após a determinação dos pontos **3**, **3e**, **4** e **4e**, aparecerão duas circunferências que correspondem às órbitas oculares e os seus respectivos centros, representados por círculos amarelos (Figura 22). Estarão liberados também no diagrama à esquerda, os demais pontos a serem demarcados.

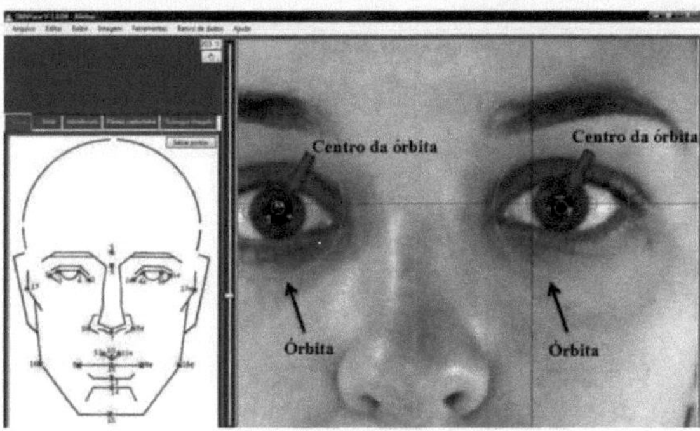

Figura 22

5. GLABELA

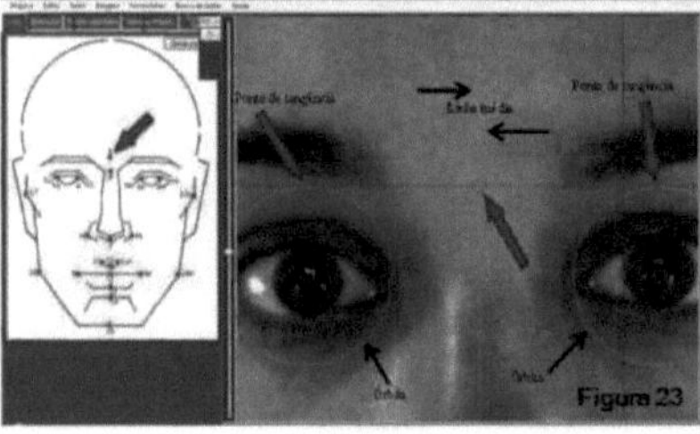
Figura 23

Descrição Fotoantropométrica

Intersecção entre a linha média orbital e a linha horizontal que tangencia o bordo superior da circunferência orbitária.

Procedimentos para a marcação do ponto

Selecionar o ponto número 5 no diagrama facial (seta vermelha Fig. 23) e dar zoom na imagem até o enquadramento da região analisada, se a resolução permitir. Deverão ser utilizadas a **linha média orbital** e a **linha horizontal** de referência para a marcação desse ponto. A linha horizontal deve ser posicionada de forma que tangencie o bordo superior das circunferências orbitárias (definidas após a marcação dos pontos irídios **3**, **3e**, **4** e **4e**). O ponto glabela deverá ser marcado na região de interseção entre elas (vide imagem ao lado).

Lembrete: Antes da determinação final de qualquer ponto, por meio da tecla "**Enter**", reduzir a imagem afim de verificar o adequado posicionamento do ponto.

6. NÁSIO

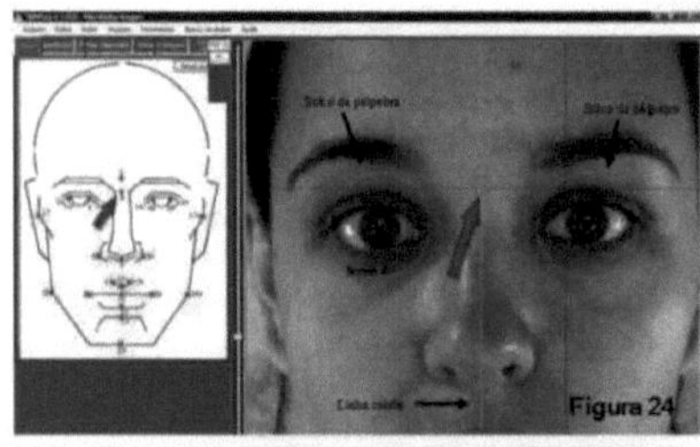
Figura 24

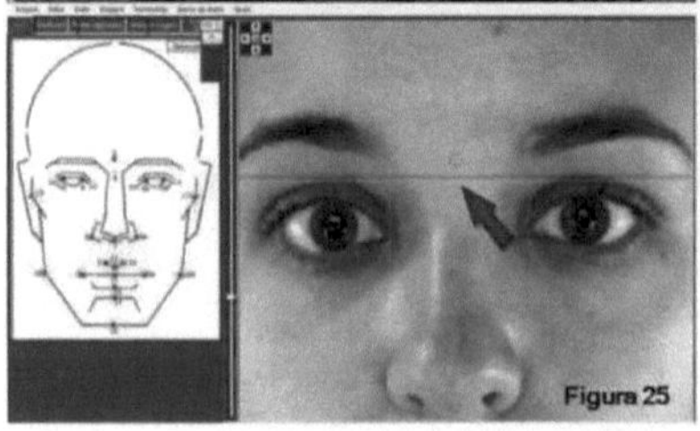
Figura 25

Descrição Fotoantropométrica

Intersecção da linha média orbital com a linha horizontal que passa pelo sulco palpebral superior.

Procedimentos para a marcação do ponto

Selecionar o ponto número 6 no diagrama facial (seta vermelha Fig. 24) e dar zoom na imagem até o enquadramento da região analisada, se a resolução permitir. Deverão ser utilizadas, a **linha média orbital** e a **linha horizontal** de referência para a marcação desse ponto. A linha horizontal deve ser posicionada de forma que tangencie a parte mais superior dos sulcos formados pelas pálpebras. O ponto násio deverá ser marcado na região de interseção entre elas. Como são dois sulcos, direito e esquerdo, quando estes estão presentes em alturas diferentes, devemos considerar a média entre as alturas dos sulcos das pálpebras. Nesse caso, deve-se inserir mais duas linhas horizontais de referência (no exemplo, linha amarela e vermelha), marcando cada sulco palpebral com uma delas. Definir então, a média entre elas com a terceira linha horizontal (no exemplo, linha verde) (Figura 25).

7. SUBNASAL

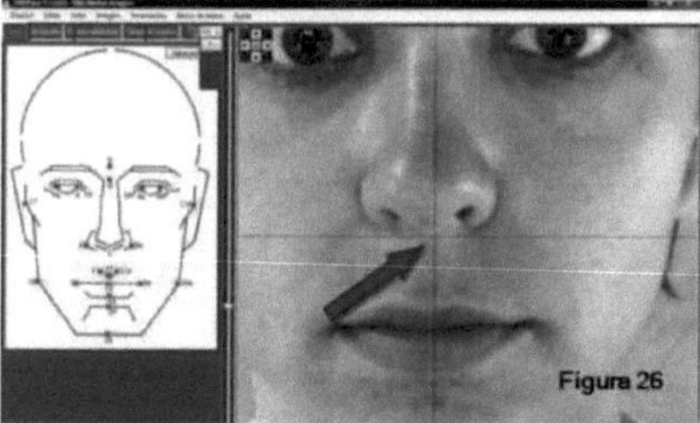
Figura 26

Descrição Fotoantropométrica

Ponto mais inferior da columela (projeção que se encontra entre as narinas).

Procedimentos para a marcação do ponto

Selecionar o ponto número 7 no diagrama facial (seta Fig. 26) e dar zoom na imagem até o enquadramento da região analisada, se a resolução permitir. Deverão ser utilizadas a **linha vertical** e a **linha horizontal** de referência para a marcação desse ponto. Essas linhas devem ser posicionadas de forma que tangenciem a parte mais inferior da projeção na base do nariz (columela). O ponto subnasal deverá ser marcado na região de interseção entre elas (vide imagem ao lado). **Não considerar a linha média orbital para a marcação desse ponto.**

8. ALAR

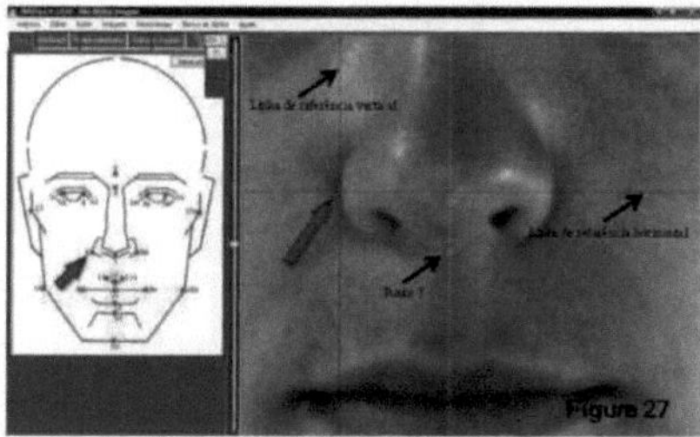
Figura 27

Descrição Fotoantropométrica

Ponto mais lateral da asa (saliência semilunar) do nariz.

Procedimentos para a marcação do ponto

Selecionar o ponto número 8 no diagrama facial (seta vermelha Fig. 27) e dar zoom na imagem até o enquadramento da região analisada, se a resolução permitir. Deverão ser utilizadas as linhas de referência para a marcação do ponto, deslocando primeiramente a **linha vertical** do lado lateral para medial do nariz e, posteriormente, a **linha horizontal**, de baixo para cima, até posiciona-las no ponto mais externo da aba do nariz. O alar deverá ser marcado na região de interseção entre as duas linhas de referência. Seguir o mesmo procedimento para marcação do ponto contralateral (**8e**).

Lembrete: Antes da determinação final de qualquer ponto, por meio da tecla "**Enter**", reduzir a imagem afim de verificar o adequado posicionamento do ponto.

9. CHELION

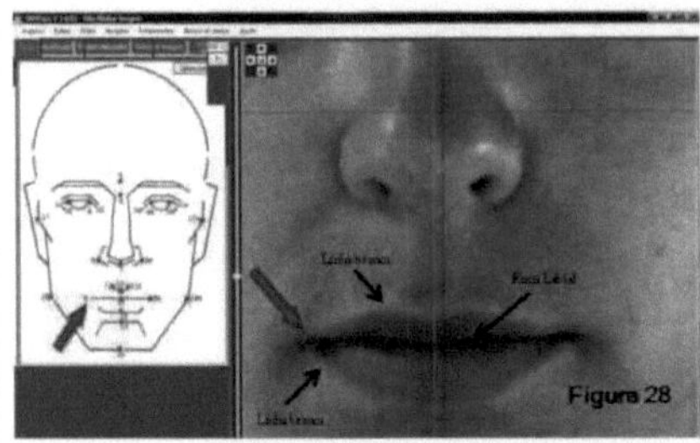
Figura 28

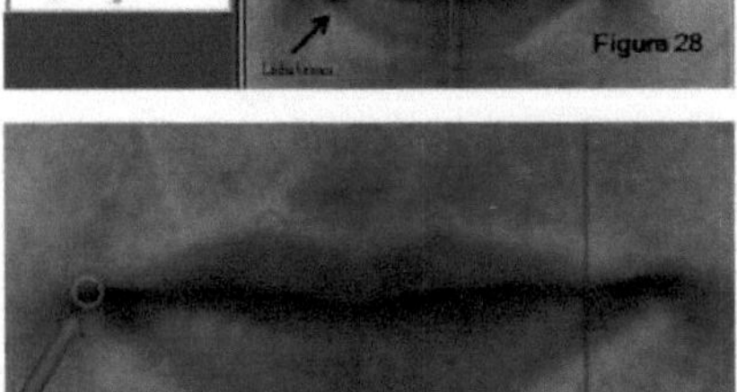
Figura 29

Descrição Fotoantropométrica

Região de encontro da linha branca (linha de transição entre a mucosa labial e a epiderme) dos lábios superior e inferior sobre a rima labial. Extensão mais lateral da linha escurecida (rima labial) formada pelo encontro dos lábios superior e inferior.

Procedimentos para a marcação do ponto

Selecionar o ponto número 9 no diagrama facial (seta vermelha Fig. 28) e dar zoom na imagem até o enquadramento da região analisada, se a resolução permitir. Podem ser utilizadas as linhas de referência para a marcação desse ponto, deslocando primeiramente a **linha vertical** do lado lateral para medial da boca e, posteriormente, a **linha horizontal**, de baixo para cima, até posiciona-las no ponto mais externo da rima labial (linha escura formada pela união do lábio superior com o lábio inferior) (Fig. 29). O chelion deverá ser marcado na região de interseção entre as duas linhas de referência. Seguir o mesmo procedimento para marcação do ponto contralateral (**9e**).

OBSERVAÇÃO - PONTO CHELION

A determinação desses pontos (**9** e **9e** - setas pretas) revelará a **linha média labial** que auxiliará a determinação dos pontos labial inferior e estômio (Figura 30).

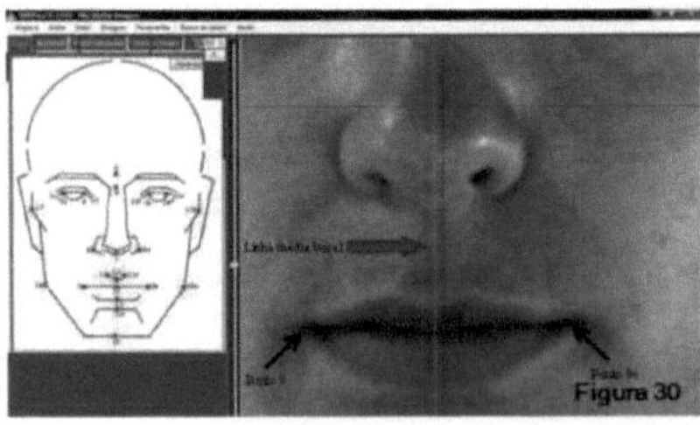
Figura 30

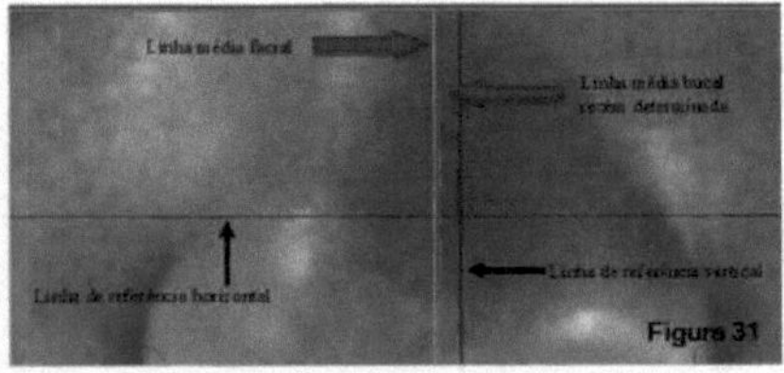
Figura 31

Esta linha é diferente da linha média orbital. No exemplo, as duas linhas médias praticamente coincidem (Figura 31), porém isto nem sempre acontece.

10. LABIAL SUPERIOR

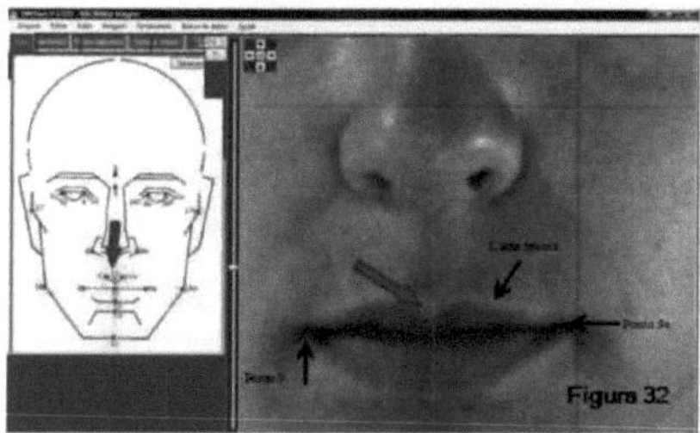
Figura 32

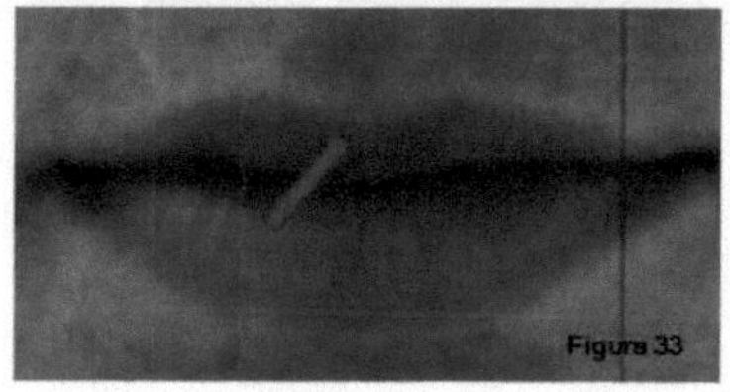
Figura 33

Descrição Fotoantropométrica

Ponto médio do lábio superior sobre a linha branca. Ponto mais inferior do arco do cupido (quando presente). Esse arco está presente no lábio superior, na região mediana e possui formato de "V".

Procedimentos para a marcação do ponto

Selecionar o ponto número 10 no diagrama facial (seta vermelha Fig. 32) e dar zoom na imagem até o enquadramento da região analisada, se a resolução permitir. Podem ser utilizadas as linhas de referência para a marcação desse ponto, deslocando primeiramente a **linha vertical** do lado lateral para medial da boca e, posteriormente, a **linha horizontal**, de baixo para cima, até posiciona-las no ponto mais inferior do ápice do "V" do arco do cupido (Fig. 33). O ponto labial superior deverá ser marcado sobre a linha de transição do vermelhão da boca com a pele circunvizinha (**linha branca**). Quando o arco do cupido não está presente, localizar o ponto mais superior do lábio. **Não considerar as linhas médias como referência.**

11. ESTÔMIO

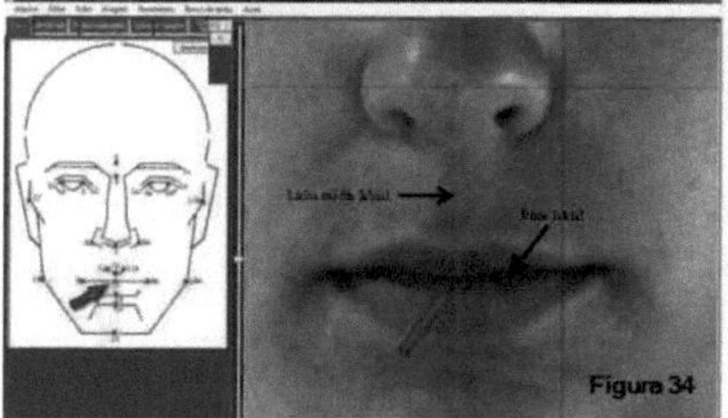
Figura 34

Descrição Fotoantropométrica

Ponto médio da rima labial (linha escura formada pela união dos lábios) de encontro ao lábio superior. Localizado medialmente aos pontos chelion direito e chelion esquerdo.

Procedimentos para a marcação do ponto

Selecionar o ponto número 12 no diagrama facial (seta vermelha Fig. 34) e dar zoom na imagem até o enquadramento da região analisada, se a resolução permitir. Deve ser utilizada a **linha média labial** como referência para a marcação desse ponto. O estômio deverá ser marcado sobre a rima labial (linha escura formada pela união dos lábios superior e inferior) no seu encontro com o lábio superior.

Lembrete: Antes da determinação de qualquer ponto, por meio da tecla "**Enter**", reduzir a imagem afim de verificar o adequado posicionamento do ponto.

12. LABIAL INFERIOR

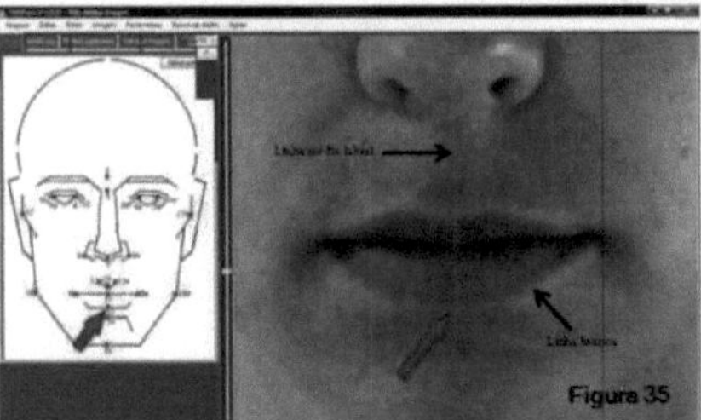

Figura 35

Descrição Fotoantropométrica

Ponto de encontro da linha média labial com o ponto mais inferior da linha branca do lábio inferior.

Procedimentos para a marcação do ponto

Selecionar o ponto número 13 no diagrama facial (seta vermelha Fig. 35) e dar zoom na imagem até o enquadramento da região analisada, se a resolução permitir. Deve ser utilizada a **linha média labial** como referência para a marcação desse ponto. O ponto labial inferior deverá ser marcado sobre a linha de transição do vermelhão da boca com a pele circunvizinha (**linha branca**) na intersecção com a linha média labial.

13. LABIOMENTAL

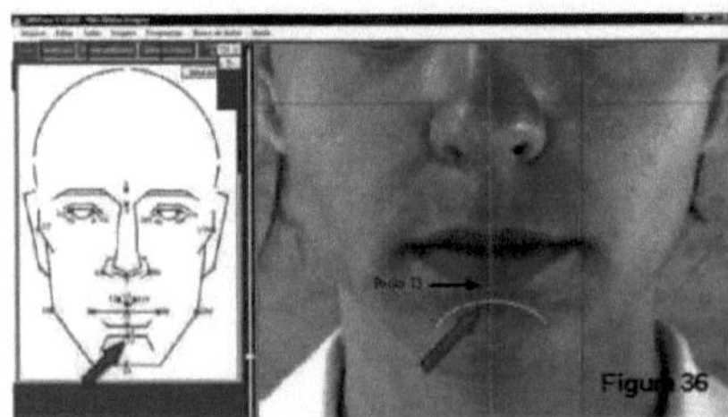

Figura 36

Descrição Fotoantropométrica

Ponto médio do sulco labiomental (linha semilunar de maior depressão entre o lábio inferior e o mento, no exemplo, representado pela linha pontilhada amarela). Visualizando da região mediana do lábio inferior até o queixo, é o ponto que marca a região de transição entre sombra (sulco labiomental) e luz (projeção do mento).

Procedimentos para a marcação do ponto

Selecionar o ponto número 14 no diagrama facial (seta vermelha Fig. 36) e dar zoom na imagem até o enquadramento da região analisada, se a resolução permitir. Deve ser utilizada a **linha média orbital** como referência para a marcação desse ponto. O ponto labiomental deverá ser marcado na intersecção da linha média orbital com o sulco labiomental, onde é possível detectar uma transição de sombra para luz, quando visualizada da região mediana do lábio inferior até o queixo.

14. GNÁTIO

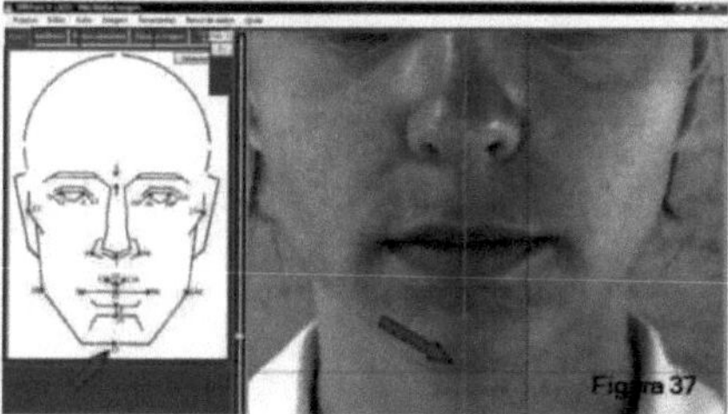
Figura 37

Descrição Fotoantropométrica

Ponto médio mais inferior do queixo. Não considerar a região de papada, quando presente.

Procedimentos para a marcação do ponto

Selecionar o ponto número 15 no diagrama facial (seta vermelha Fig. 37) e dar zoom na imagem até o enquadramento da região analisada, se a resolução permitir. Quando o queixo não apresenta ponto mais inferior, por possuir uma forma mais retilínea, deve ser utilizada a **linha média orbital** como referência para a marcação desse ponto. Quando há uma projeção maior (notória o suficiente para dizer que é uma característica pessoal) e, sendo possível a definição de um ponto mais inferior, a linha média orbital não deve ser considerada.

15. GÔNIO

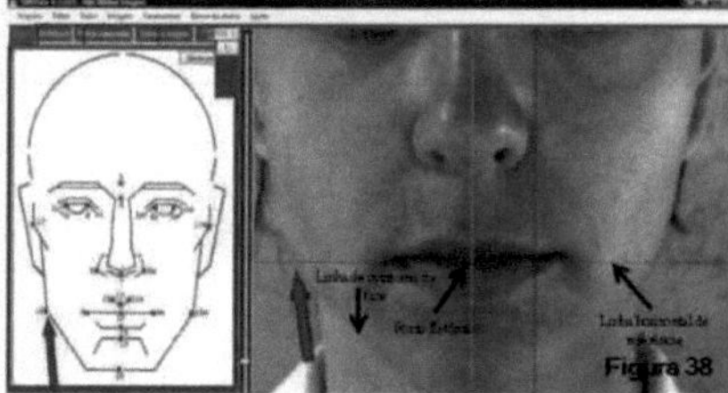
Figura 38

Descrição Fotoantropométrica

Ponto mais lateral onde a linha horizontal de referência passa pelo ponto estômio e cruza a linha de contorno da face.

Procedimentos para a marcação do ponto

Selecionar o ponto número 16 no diagrama facial (seta vermelha Fig. 38) e dar zoom na imagem até o enquadramento da região analisada, se a resolução permitir. Deve ser utilizada a **linha horizontal** como referência para a marcação desse ponto. O gônio deverá ser marcado no ponto de tangência da linha horizontal de referência, passando pelo estômio, com o contorno da face. Seguir o mesmo procedimento para marcação do ponto contralateral (**16e**).

16. ZÍGIO

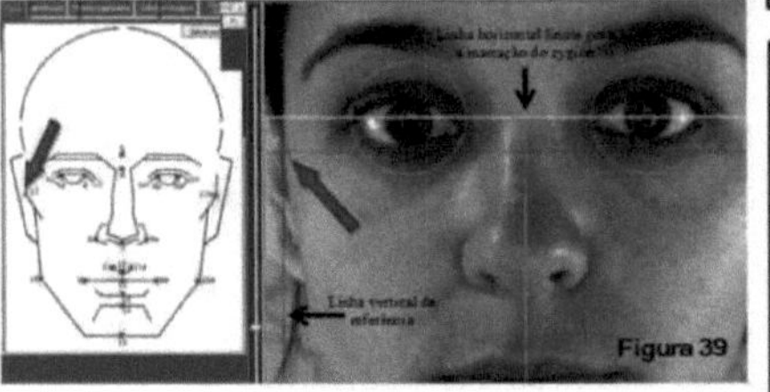
Figura 39

Descrição Fotoantropométrica

Ponto mais lateral da face (maior largura) do osso zigomático, na região da maçã do rosto.

Procedimentos para a marcação do ponto

Selecionar o ponto número 17 no diagrama facial (seta vermelha Fig. 39) e dar zoom na imagem até o enquadramento da região analisada, se a resolução permitir. Deverão ser utilizadas linhas de referência para a marcação do ponto, deslocando primeiramente a **linha vertical** do lado lateral para medial da face e, posteriormente, a **linha horizontal**, de baixo para cima, até posiciona-las na região mais proeminente (de maior largura) da face. O zígio deverá ser marcado na região de interseção entre elas (vide figura ao lado). Seguir o mesmo procedimento para a marcação do ponto contralateral (**17e**).

Atenção: A marcação deste ponto é independente do mesmo ponto contralateral, ou seja, ambos não necessitam ter o mesmo plano horizontal de referência. Ambos os pontos devem ter, como limite vertical, uma linha horizontal que passa pelo centro da órbita.

Appendix B - Data resulting from the descriptive statistics for each specific point.

Alar	Distance in X		Y distance		Euclidean distance	
	Phase 1	Phase 2	Phase 1	Phase 2	Phase 1	Phase 2
Maximum	4,490	2,556	9,278	5,677	9,293	5,853
Q3	1,237	0,728	3,411	1,856	3,696	1,976
Average	0,859	0,497	2,332	1,371	2,660	1,550
Median	0,671	0,318	1,994	1,187	2,312	1,373
Q1	0,266	0,141	0,750	0,490	1,395	0,754
Minimum	0,011	0,000	0,019	0,000	0,182	0,000
Standard Deviation	0,758	0,475	1,871	1,131	1,780	1,107
Coefficient of variation	0,883	0,956	0,803	0,825	0,669	0,714
Chelion	Distance in X		Y distance		Euclidean distance	
	Phase 1	Phase 2	Phase 1	Phase 2	Phase 1	Phase 2
Maximum	9,275	9,906	2,694	4,825	9,571	9,907
Q3	3,091	3,511	0,946	1,304	3,258	3,837
Average	2,149	2,507	0,663	0,960	2,352	2,835
Median	1,776	2,148	0,511	0,734	1,968	2,475
Q1	0,698	0,879	0,270	0,346	0,972	1,282
Minimum	0,003	0,000	0,008	0,000	0,043	0,000
Standard Deviation	1,806	2,144	0,544	0,904	1,756	2,140
Coefficient of variation	0,841	0,855	0,821	0,942	0,747	0,755
Ectocanthion	Distance in X		Y distance		Euclidean distance	
	Phase 1	Phase 2	Phase 1	Phase 2	Phase 1	Phase 2
Maximum	11,395	11,050	4,771	7,467	11,566	11,831
Q3	5,141	3,467	1,728	1,905	5,373	3,904
Average	3,751	2,418	1,183	1,329	4,055	2,994
Median	3,493	2,053	0,984	1,071	3,603	2,612
Q1	2,009	0,874	0,479	0,467	2,347	1,518
Minimum	0,045	0,026	0,015	0,010	0,198	0,087
Standard Deviation	2,280	1,959	0,859	1,168	2,226	1,961
Coefficient of variation	0,608	0,810	0,726	0,879	0,549	0,655
Endocanthion	Distance in X		Y distance		Euclidean distance	
	Phase 1	Phase 2	Phase 1	Phase 2	Phase 1	Phase 2

Maximum	22,707	6,743	2,764	4,506	22,866	6,783
Q3	2,153	1,587	1,220	1,391	2,583	2,082
Average	1,763	1,229	0,852	0,965	2,125	1,730
Median	1,250	0,889	0,724	0,753	1,684	1,483
Q1	0,546	0,409	0,338	0,315	0,969	0,806
Minimum	0,002	0,000	0,012	0,010	0,133	0,038
Standard Deviation	2,269	1,244	0,643	0,829	2,208	1,297
Coefficient of variation	1,287	1,012	0,755	0,859	1,039	0,749
Stomach	Distance in X		Y distance		Euclidean distance	
	Phase 1	Phase 2	Phase 1	Phase 2	Phase 1	Phase 2
Maximum	12,674	6,693	31,975	2,577	32,007	6,718
Q3	2,528	2,906	1,027	0,942	3,026	3,028
Average	1,886	1,926	1,366	0,705	2,700	2,190
Median	1,482	1,557	0,593	0,609	1,734	1,858
Q1	0,782	0,585	0,340	0,278	0,970	1,087
Minimum	0,007	0,006	0,034	0,021	0,154	0,038
Standard Deviation	1,731	1,633	3,654	0,520	3,802	1,531
Coefficient of variation	0,918	0,848	2,674	0,739	1,408	0,699
Glabella	Distance in X		Y distance		Euclidean distance	
	Phase 1	Phase 2	Phase 1	Phase 2	Phase 1	Phase 2
Maximum	16,256	3,581	38,609	7,065	38,678	7,921
Q3	4,466	1,256	17,008	2,452	17,653	2,598
Average	3,183	0,864	13,581	1,750	14,316	2,091
Median	2,728	0,686	12,906	1,481	13,567	1,800
Q1	1,446	0,360	8,562	0,698	9,487	1,146
Minimum	0,169	0,006	0,936	0,009	1,972	0,192
Standard Deviation	2,483	0,696	7,558	1,433	7,266	1,402
Coefficient of variation	0,780	0,805	0,557	0,819	0,508	0,671
Gnatio	Distance in X		Y distance		Euclidean distance	
	Phase 1	Phase 2	Phase 1	Phase 2	Phase 1	Phase 2
Maximum	10,220	16,574	4,061	2,721	10,255	16,581
Q3	3,830	3,917	1,357	0,888	4,083	3,969
Average	2,663	2,867	0,999	0,660	3,033	3,072
Median	2,124	2,057	0,844	0,598	2,669	2,280
Q1	1,191	0,703	0,424	0,281	1,560	1,206
Minimum	0,023	0,000	0,001	0,000	0,147	0,000
Standard Deviation	2,105	3,007	0,806	0,493	1,990	2,914
Coefficient of variation	0,790	1,049	0,807	0,747	0,656	0,948
Ionian	Distance in X		Y distance		Distance Euclidean	
	Phase 1	Phase 2	Phase 1	Phase 2	Phase 1	Phase 2
Maximum	25,663	7,529	70,561	3,443	75,083	7,573
Q3	9,692	1,332	22,643	1,194	24,854	1,778
Average	7,077	1,003	16,843	0,848	18,418	1,431
Median	6,090	0,782	13,438	0,687	14,667	1,210
Q1	3,051	0,435	6,616	0,398	7,604	0,792
Minimum	0,154	0,013	0,140	0,030	0,898	0,244
Standard Deviation	5,264	0,909	13,788	0,651	14,571	0,961
Coefficient of variation	0,744	0,906	0,819	0,768	0,791	0,672
Lateral Iridium	Distance in X		Y distance		Euclidean distance	
	Phase 1	Phase 2	Phase 1	Phase 2	Phase 1	Phase 2
Maximum	3,203	2,476	4,667	3,117	4,668	3,125
Q3	0,936	0,711	1,673	1,206	1,910	1,407
Average	0,697	0,495	1,155	0,830	1,473	1,062
Median	0,556	0,400	0,999	0,641	1,304	0,926
Q1	0,263	0,199	0,438	0,344	0,837	0,582
Minimum	0,003	0,011	0,013	0,002	0,132	0,075
Standard Deviation	0,631	0,389	0,867	0,659	0,893	0,624
Coefficient of variation	0,906	0,786	0,751	0,794	0,606	0,588
Medial Iridium	Distance in X		Y distance		Euclidean distance	
	Phase 1	Phase 2	Phase 1	Phase 2	Phase 1	Phase2
Maximum	18,600	1,743	17,411	3,496	25,477	3,496

Q3	0,923	0,645	1,368	1,136	1,730	1,322
Average	0,773	0,450	1,128	0,833	1,472	1,023
Median	0,477	0,353	0,814	0,681	1,108	0,925
Q1	0,207	0,178	0,393	0,319	0,680	0,505
Minimum	0,012	0,004	0,009	0,004	0,059	0,080
Standard Deviation	1,533	0,362	1,517	0,669	2,086	0,654
Coefficient of variation	1,984	0,806	1,346	0,803	1,417	0,640

Lower lip	Distance in X		Y distance		Euclidean distance	
	Phase 1	Phase 2	Phase 1	Phase 2	Phase 1	Phase 2
Maximum	10,583	6,693	6,490	13,723	10,641	14,051
Q3	2,662	2,627	2,478	2,167	3,776	3,702
Average	2,070	1,875	1,718	1,688	2,993	2,854
Median	1,894	1,413	1,470	1,326	2,500	2,441
Q1	0,897	0,558	0,527	0,535	1,810	1,636
Minimum	0,040	0,000	0,046	0,000	0,115	0,000
Standard Deviation	1,757	1,627	1,434	1,784	1,845	2,006
Coefficient of variation	0,849	0,868	0,835	1,056	0,616	0,703

Upper lip	Distance in X		Y distance		Euclidean distance	
	Phase 1	Phase 2	Phase 1	Phase 2	Phase 1	Phase 2
Maximum	14,765	6,948	18,577	7,029	18,726	7,138
Q3	2,473	1,548	5,171	2,614	5,912	3,359
Average	2,004	1,294	3,737	1,867	4,634	2,540
Median	1,478	0,914	2,766	1,647	3,914	2,096
Q1	0,895	0,464	1,419	0,792	2,042	1,460
Minimum	0,142	0,022	0,008	0,004	0,238	0,273
Standard Deviation	1,946	1,264	3,465	1,390	3,501	1,491
Coefficient of variation	0,971	0,977	0,927	0,744	0,755	0,587

Labiomental	Distance in X		Y distance		Euclidean distance	
	Phase 1	Phase 2	Phase 1	Phase 2	Phase 1	Phase 2
Maximum	9,827	13,569	17,914	14,065	18,137	15,642
Q3	3,424	2,734	8,506	7,699	9,758	8,828
Average	2,542	2,115	5,588	5,248	6,668	6,092
Median	1,917	1,388	3,978	5,135	5,633	6,090
Q1	0,939	0,606	1,664	2,124	2,920	3,006
Minimum	0,105	0,000	0,018	0,000	0,352	0,000
Standard Deviation	2,240	2,301	4,807	3,743	4,613	3,761
Coefficient of variation	0,881	1,088	0,860	0,713	0,692	0,617

Násio	Distance in X		Y distance		Euclidean distance	
	Phase 1	Phase 2	Phase 1	Phase 2	Phase 1	Phase 2
Maximum	16,051	3,581	25,940	3,424	26,649	3,598
Q3	3,859	1,311	12,085	1,022	12,103	1,680
Average	2,734	0,908	7,229	0,761	8,364	1,340
Median	2,265	0,726	5,540	0,540	6,642	1,303
Q1	1,133	0,370	2,239	0,259	4,312	0,793
Minimum	0,050	0,003	0,018	0,007	0,534	0,175
Standard Deviation	2,281	0,715	6,122	0,689	5,686	0,767
Coefficient of variation	0,835	0,788	0,847	0,905	0,680	0,572

Subnasal	Distance in X		Y distance		Euclidean distance	
	Phase 1	Phase 2	Phase 1	Phase 2	Phase 1	Phase 2
Maximum	15,716	5,160	11,124	4,910	19,255	5,727
Q3	1,775	1,977	1,792	1,401	2,571	2,551
Average	1,412	1,395	1,394	0,996	2,217	1,924
Median	0,928	1,179	1,005	0,592	1,863	1,620
Q1	0,382	0,486	0,500	0,365	1,057	0,906
Minimum	0,030	0,016	0,001	0,006	0,074	0,071
Standard Deviation	1,900	1,169	1,612	0,951	2,284	1,225
Coefficient of variation	1,345	0,838	1,156	0,955	1,030	0,637

Zygian	Distance in X		Y distance		Euclidean distance	
	Phase 1	Phase 2	Phase 1	Phase 2	Phase 1	Phase 2
Maximum	12,501	4,875	48,829	46,494	48,840	46,494

Q3	3,336	1,427	15,481	8,752	15,683	8,857
Average	2,616	0,968	11,499	6,671	12,129	6,881
Median	1,989	0,781	9,663	5,386	10,550	5,455
Q1	1,065	0,380	5,401	2,545	6,149	2,791
Minimum	0,016	0,006	0,092	0,037	0,208	0,047
Standard Deviation	2,218	0,761	8,409	6,326	8,218	6,219
Coefficient of variation	0,848	0,786	0,731	0,948	0,678	0,904

Annex A - Opinion of the Research Ethics Committee

FACULDADE DE ODONTOLOGIA DE RIBEIRÃO PRETO/ FORP/ USP

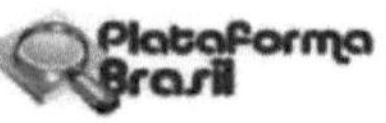

PARECER CONSUBSTANCIADO DO CEP

DADOS DO PROJETO DE PESQUISA

Título da Pesquisa: PROPOSTA DE MÉTODO DE ADEQUAÇÃO DOS PONTOS DE REFERÊNCIA DA ANTROPOMETRIA CRANIOFACIAL PARA EMPREGO EM EXAMES FACIAIS EM FOTOGRAFIAS FRONTAIS: RESULTADOS PRELIMINARES

Pesquisador: Marta Regina Pinheiro Flores

Área Temática:

Versão: 4

CAAE: 17902713.7.0000.5419

Instituição Proponente: Universidade de Sao Paulo

Patrocinador Principal: Financiamento Próprio

DADOS DO PARECER

Número do Parecer: 619.630

Apresentação do Projeto:

Os exames de Identificação Facial baseiam-se na premissa de que não existem dois indivíduos com a mesma constituição anatômica. O trabalho tem como objetivo propor um método de análise facial voltado ao exame de fotografias em norma frontal e avaliar quais são os pontos cefalométricos que apresentam maior e menor variabilidade de aferição.

O estudo será dividido em duas etapas. A primeira consistirá na sistematização da técnica de exame facial exclusivamente baseado em fotografias frontais. A segunda fase será experimental, onde cinco examinadores analisarão 13 imagens de um banco de dados de indivíduos adultos, de ambos os sexos, todos fotografados em norma frontal. Como resultado espera-se o aprimoramento da técnica de exame facial em norma frontal sobre imagens fotográficas, assim como o robustecimento dos exames realizados na prática pericial.

Objetivo da Pesquisa:

Propor uma metodologia de normalização dos pontos cefalométricos para a realização de exames faciais baseados em imagens fotográficas, bem como avaliar quais são os pontos cefalométricos que apresentam maior e menor variabilidade de aferição, dentro da metodologia proposta.

Situação do Parecer:

Aprovado

Necessita Apreciação da CONEP:

Não

Considerações Finais a critério do CEP:

Conforme deliberado na 162ª R.E. do CEP.

Endereço: Avenida do Café s/nº
Bairro: Monte Alegre **CEP:** 14.040-904
UF: SP **Município:** RIBEIRAO PRETO
Telefone: (16)3602-0251 **Fax:** (16)3602-4102 **E-mail:** cep@forp.usp.br

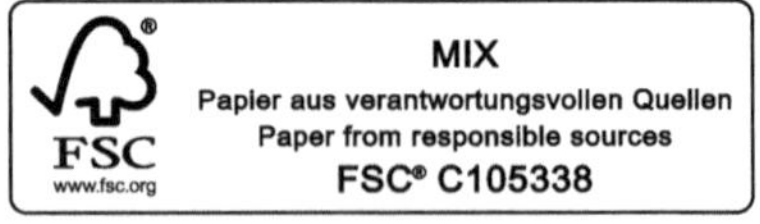

Printed by Books on Demand GmbH, Norderstedt / Germany